What People Are Saying About

ReInventing Cool

Cold thermogenesis through whole body cryotherapy is a powerful practice, lasting just 3 minutes, yet offering a cascade of health benefits. This method, grounded in our past where our ancestors thrived in cold environments, has now been shown by solid research to boost metabolism, regulate blood glucose, reduce inflammation, and improve sleep and recovery. Its potential extends to combating certain cancers and promoting longevity. As someone who competed in Ironman triathlons and experienced extensive cold exposure, I can attest to the lasting metabolic advantages. Whole body cryotherapy is not just a modern wellness trend; it's a scientifically backed approach to enhancing physical and mental performance.

Ben Greenfield, biohacker, health consultant, and *New York Times* bestselling author of numerous books, including *Beyond Training* and *Boundless*

I'm very glad and excited about *ReInventing Cool*. Whole body cryotherapy is a long-proven treatment still not fully understood by the public. Maria and Antra are both renowned wellness industry pioneers, aware of the needs of the fast-growing market, not only with regard to education on safety and efficacy. They show and explain all relevant touchpoints and open the doors to understanding the full power of this twenty-first-century lifestyle treatment. A must-read for everybody interested in living a healthy and happy life.

Rainer Bolsinger, Chair of Global Wellness Institute Cryotherapy Initiative

T0300780

This book is what the cryotherapy and wellness world has desperately needed. As the industry continues to expand, more knowledge and research is in demand, and this is the perfect answer to that. This resource will help this evolving industry to continue to grow.

Kelly Carden, Founder of Cryotherapy Industry National Association

Over the last decade, whole body cryotherapy has evolved from a niche, somewhat esoteric practice to a widely sought-after therapy by millions. This rapid expansion, however, has given rise to numerous myths and misunderstandings. *ReInventing Cool* arrives at a pivotal moment, offering invaluable insights for wellness center proprietors to better navigate their industry. It also helps clients and potential customers with more grounded expectations and adequate preparation. We at NEXT Wellness commend the collaborative effort of two esteemed figures in the field — a seasoned treatment provider and a renowned business coach and educator — for authoring a seminal work that promises to further empower individuals in the pursuit of health and longevity.

Jay Houston, co-CEO of NEXT Wellness, Inc. 5000

Finally, there is a resource to help! As a cryotherapy center owner, I've witnessed firsthand the prevalent misconceptions surrounding cryotherapy. It isn't just about extreme cold; it's a holistic wellness solution. In the process of building our business, we had to bridge the gap between perception and reality and put a lot of effort into making users not only engage but also understand the science behind cryotherapy. I wish we had *ReInventing Cool* in our hands when we first started! The book goes into important detail in an easy-to-read way and will

be a great guide to all who want to better understand why to use cold, when, and how.
Paul Hooten, owner of Ultra Cryo & Recovery

Maria and Antra are true innovators in the cold therapy space with a passion for educating and giving practical yet proven no-nonsense advice. As an owner of a wellness clinic that provides multiple types of cold therapy, I can attest that whole body cryotherapy is, hands down, the most beneficial service in our portfolio and a crucial component of a holistic drug-free longevity routine. Our clients have given us countless testimonials recounting the benefits they have personally experienced, including improved mobility, decreased pain and inflammation, increased energy, improved mood, and better sleep. This book provides a roadmap on how to incorporate whole-body cryotherapy to achieve these results.
Mike Schwarz, founder of CoolCRYO

Attitudes to health are changing, and Maria and Antra have written this brilliant guide on the life-changing benefits of cryotherapy. I work and work out harder than I've ever done. Without cryotherapy being part of my recovery, it just wouldn't be possible. You have to try it!
Melanie Chisholm, aka Mel C of the Spice Girls

I didn't like the cold ... I didn't think I liked the cold ... I love the cold. Through various points over the last 10 years cryotherapy has helped me recover better after training, helped get me back training during darker spells when I lost the discipline to show up, manage weight and blood sugar, and during some pretty difficult times given me a lift mentally which has allowed me to start putting the pieces back together. When I find myself in a slump if I've fallen out of a routine where I no longer use the cold regularly it's the cold I return to so as I can begin reclaiming my life. Everyone who uses the cold has a reason — injury, energy, longevity, mood — whatever the reason, all the other benefits come with it and unlike most things the benefits are cumulative, they don't begin to wane with regular use — quite the opposite. Now you also have the addition of targeted cryo for muscle soreness/injury, cryo facials (apparently five in a row is equivalent to a facelift!) and cryo slimming. I personally enjoy contrast therapy — using the infrared sauna in between rounds of cold. LondonCryo is literally a sanctuary for those seeking to feel as good as can be.

Now that we have *ReInventing Cool* by Maria and Antra, we can all understand why our ancestors turned to cold for its powerful impact on their health and why it's the way forward to reap all the benefits I've experienced firsthand.

Stephen Manderson, aka Professor Green

ReInventing Cool

How to Make COLD Your Best Ally against Inflammation, Pain, and Aging

Maria Ensabella & Antra Getzoff

BOOKS

London, UK
Washington, DC, USA

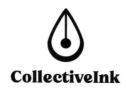

CollectiveInk

First published by O-Books, 2025
O-Books is an imprint of Collective Ink Ltd.,
Unit 11, Shepperton House, 89 Shepperton Road, London, N1 3DF
office@collectiveinkbooks.com
www.collectiveinkbooks.com
www.o-books.com

For distributor details and how to order please visit the 'Ordering' section on our website.

Text copyright: Maria Ensabella & Antra Getzoff, 2024

ISBN: 978 1 80341 757 8
978 1 80341 775 2 (ebook)
Library of Congress Control Number: 2024930438

A CIP catalogue record for this book is available from the British Library.

Design: Lapiz Digital Services

UK: Printed and bound by CPI Group (UK) Ltd, Croydon, CR0 4YY
Printed in North America by CPI GPS partners

The authors of this book do not dispense medical advice or
prescribe the use of any technique as a form of treatment for
physical, emotional, or medical problems without the advice of a
physician, either directly or indirectly. The intent of the authors
is only to offer information of a general nature to help you in
your quest for emotional and spiritual well-being. In the event
you use any of the information in this book for yourself, which is
your constitutional right, the authors and the publisher assume no
responsibility for your actions.

We operate a distinctive and ethical publishing philosophy in
all areas of our business, from our global network of authors to
production and worldwide distribution.

Contents

How Cold Shaped Our Lives and May Change Yours Too

Behind every beginning, there is a story. Like many others, we were not seeking cryotherapy. We bumped into it and were curious to try. But once we did, there was no way back — the first encounter turned into love that grew strong and made us both not only continue with treatments but also change our careers and turn into ambassadors of the many powers of cold. In a nutshell...

Hello, I am Maria Ensabella!

Although southern Italian by ethnicity, I grew up in Melbourne, Australia. Maybe that's why the cultural perspective of getting married and having children, then focusing on being a good housewife and slowly gaining weight in the process of feeding the family did not appeal. I vividly remember the moment when I, 17 at the time, made myself a promise to never end up suffering from obesity and diabetes like many women in my vicinity.

What started with group classes and weight training at the local gym and deliberately healthy meals requested from my mother grew into even more passion for health and fitness, especially running, after moving to London 15 years later. Not long after giving birth to a baby girl at a not-so-young age there came the first completed marathon, followed by many more long-distance races that emphasized the importance of recuperation.

I was preparing for the New York marathon when I heard the great American motivational speaker and biohacking pioneer Tony Robbins talk about cryotherapy. He was crediting cold exposures for speedier recovery from his multi-hour stage performances. Right there, in NYC, inspired by Tony, I tried whole body cryotherapy for the first time. Relief from the stress, jetlag, and muscle soreness was immediate. It felt game changing. I did more treatments while in the United States, then in Sydney and Melbourne, but there was no way to continue after returning home to the UK. Sadly, London had no offer.

Fascinated by the physical and mental uplift I received from whole body cryotherapy and wanting to keep adding to my own life as well as to give others the chance to experience the benefits, I gave up my job as an insolvency accountant and, supported by my partner, launched LondonCryo. The first center opened in 2016. In the moment of writing these lines, we have three prime locations offering a range of leading wellness treatments, but there will be more. Seeing my clients from celebrities to young athletes, busy professionals and ageless grandmothers perform, feel, and look better is incredibly rewarding. I *love* my new career.

Interestingly, I also got a chance to give back to the man who inspired my becoming a wellness entrepreneur. I was invited to take part in setting up a recovery suite for Tony Robbins at one of his shows in London.

Hey there, I'm Antra Getzoff!

I grew up and built a career in management, training, and consulting in Latvia. It is possible that not much would have changed to date if it was not for cryotherapy. Cold, quite literally, changed my life ... twice.

As a little girl, I could never stand still. My mother says she would always recognize me in the distance because of my nonstop bouncing. The bottomless supply of energy had to be funneled into something, and my parents chose dancing. They took me to my first dance class when I was just 4.

Even after leaving the dance floor to build a career and a family, there were always fitness classes, yoga, Nordic walking, hiking, biking, skiing, nutritious home-made meals, and experiments with supplementation. But wellness was a passion, not a profession, and cold was never part of the routine. As it is for many people, even chilly showers did not feel appealing enough to commit to.

January of 2010 came with a spontaneous decision to leave the 250-person company that I had been running for the last 4 years through the stresses and hardships of the financial crisis. Walking out was an "I will never have another boss in my life" moment. Agitated, physically and emotionally drained, and sleepless, I came across an ad for a whole body cryotherapy special. The promise and the deal were too good not to try. The first ten sessions turned into ten more because the post-treatment endorphins were exactly what my exhausted body needed.

For one of my visits to the cryotherapy center, I brought along a visiting friend. This accidental introduction of an American man to extreme cold turned my life upside down in the most unexpected way. A few months later I landed in San Francisco, California to become one of the first cryotherapy entrepreneurs in the United States and the "original gangsters" of this now booming industry.

Since arriving in the USA more than a decade ago, I have helped hundreds of businesses incorporate cryotherapy into their offerings, and nothing warms my heart more than seeing them open new locations and hearing the amazing recovery stories of their clients.

Collectively, we have helped more than a million people get pain-free and live their lives to the fullest again. What could be better than that?

Hello, reader!

If this book has gotten into your hands, it is likely that you, like us, are a believer in holistic drug-free wellness as a way of life rather than a short-term project to reach some health, performance, or appearance goal. If so, we are excited to become your sparring partner. If not, we may be able to make you see well-being in a slightly different light and join the growing worldwide movement.

We have been wellness entrepreneurs for years, but, first and foremost, we remain healthy lifestyle enthusiasts, walking the walk and reaping the benefits. Discovering COLD not as an unwanted weather condition but as a super-powerful health booster has shaped our lives more than any other approach.

Hard to embrace at first, cold may well be the world's best-kept secret, not only against inflammation and pain, but also to conquer chronic stress, lack of energy and motivation, depressive mood, poor sleep, and biological aging, especially when the entire body gets exposed to it at once. Come and see for yourself! Join us on a journey of reinventing cool!

We have written this book to help you see cold with new eyes, putting to work our own experiences and feedback from hundreds of thousands of clients whom we and our fellow cryotherapy afficionados have collectively served.

This is *not* a digest of the latest research in the field, although you will see numerous references to clinical studies performed to date.

This is *not* a textbook, although we believe you will learn a thing or two regardless of your relationship with cryotherapy.

Most importantly, this should *not* be seen as professional advice on how to lessen symptoms of any medical condition, although you will find examples of substantial health improvements thanks to whole body cold.

The purpose of this practical guide is to help you use low temperatures safely, effectively, and joyfully, whether you are a team member of a gym, wellness center, or spa with cryotherapy on the menu, are thinking of starting a business that offers cryotherapy, are a client of such a business, or are bracing yourself to try cryotherapy for the first time.

In Chapter 1, we explain the often neglected yet essential differences between various types of cold applications and narrow our focus down to the main topic of this book – Whole Body Cryotherapy or WBC.

Chapter 2 describes its working mechanisms.

Chapter 3 reveals the property of whole body cryo that makes it as multifaceted as it is in terms of applications and benefits.

Chapter 4 summarizes the research findings to date and shows why in most countries whole body cryotherapy is not seen as a medical procedure.

Chapter 5 discusses the considerations to establish the optimal dose of cryotherapy depending on the goal.

Chapter 6 is dedicated to customization of the cold treatment regimen, because in cryotherapy, one size cannot fit all.

Chapter 7 puts cryotherapy in the broader context of preventive care and biohacking.

Throughout the text, you will find brief case studies to illustrate the power of low-temperature whole body cold and links to various additional resources to study cryotherapy in more depth. This is just the beginning. So, buckle up and enjoy the ride. Making the "impossible" happen personally or professionally may be easier than you think.

Yours truly,

Maria Ensabella and Antra Getzoff

Introduction

From Sick Care to Self-Care: The Tides Are Turning

Before we get into discussing whole body cryotherapy as one of the ways of improving well-being naturally through mobilizing the body's every cell and process, let us mention just a few facts demonstrating why the time to do so is NOW.

Despite mind-blowing technological advancements in almost every field impacting our lives, including medical care, statistics show a continuous and steep increase in the numbers of people suffering from pain, obesity, and depression.

Impacted by the recent pandemic and a level of drug abuse that is more massive than ever, many countries are experiencing "a dramatic fall" in life expectancy, the largest in 100 years. A 2021 report from the US National Center for Health Statistics shows a drop of 3 years in just 24 months. The reason for this was not the virus itself but the population's overall health, too bad to withstand challenges like Covid-19. Following are some sample statistics.

According to a 2015 publication by the US National Institutes of Health, 126 million American adults (more than 55%) had experienced some type of pain in the last 3 months. 40 million of them called their pain levels severe; 25.3 million lived in pain daily.

Based on data presented by the World Health Organization, the number of obese people worldwide has tripled in less than 50 years. In the USA, the percentage grew from 30.5% to 41.9% in less than a decade.

The Anxiety and Depression Association of America reports that 1 in 5 adults experience at least one major depressive disorder at some point in their lives, and the rate is growing fastest among adolescents, while suicide has become one of the leading causes of death.

At least 70% of all visits to a physician result in some form of drug therapy, driving prescription medication expenditure per capita higher and higher. As most drugs mask symptoms rather than address the cause, the development of chronic conditions remains on the rise.

Ironically, going through the pandemic became a turning point in many people's attitudes towards their own health. With less trust in the almightiness of medical care, often referred to as "sick care" due to its reactive nature, people have now started taking more responsibility and making better choices. The tides are turning. We are witnessing a big public interest shift from drug-based solutions to lifestyle adjustments and therapies boosting the immune system, preventing illness, and promoting self-healing, including exposing the body to low temperatures. This trend will likely only build in strength in the years to come.

Amid the rapidly growing popularity of cold therapies, whole body cryotherapy as the most powerful of them is getting under the radar of more and more policymakers, governments, educational institutions, and businesses. Cryotherapy is now offered not only in sports facilities and narrowly specialized rehabilitation or wellness centers. It has made its way into clinics, spas and med spas, hotels, office buildings, and even public facilities such as airports. The growing interest means there is a need for spreading knowledge to better equip current and future service providers and users alike.

Of course, wellness is the practice of healthy habits, and cryotherapy or any other nature-based therapy is not a magic wand. It cannot be seen as an isolated way to energize, heal, cure, or slim down, but, as an add-on to exercise, nutrition, hydration, sleep, and mental hygiene, it can be a powerful tool in the hands of a skilled and committed person to awaken the body for the best performance it is capable of and was built to rely on. The "inner doctor" resides within all of us and is stronger than we dare to believe.

In our lives, out of all the therapies enhancing the body's resilience and performance naturally, whole body cryotherapy has been, hands down, the biggest game changer. Once discovered, it remains both the catalyst and the bedrock of our health and wellness journeys. Hence this book as our experience-based guide to the best cryotherapy practices and to treatment protocols that have been proven to deliver results.

Chapter 1

The Many Faces of Cold and the One That We Are Only Discovering Now

The use of cold as a therapeutic agent has a long and colorful history. The Edwin Smith Papyrus, the most ancient medical text known, dated 3500 B.C., made numerous references to the use of cold as therapy. Baron de Larrey, a French army surgeon during Napoleon's Russian campaign, packed the limbs in ice prior to amputations to render the procedures painless. In the early twentieth century, a neurosurgeon, Temple Fay, pioneered "human refrigeration" as a treatment for malignancies and head injuries.

— Excerpt from an article by H. Wang and colleagues, "Cold as a Therapeutic Agent." Published in *History of Neurosurgery* on February 17, 2006

What we have known for centuries

Every trend has an origin, no matter how new or innovative it may seem. Most health-enhancing therapies of today can be traced throughout history, improving as knowledge gets acquired and technology evolves.

Localized cold (water, ice) applications but also whole-body immersions to strengthen the immune system, reduce inflammation and swelling, and minimize pain have been used for millennia.

The term *cryotherapy* is not new, either. It comes from the ancient Greek words *kruos* (ice, icy cold, chill, frost) and *therapeuo* (cure) and covers everything from an ice pack on a swollen joint to whole-body plunges and beyond. For this reason, it is possible that two people actively discussing cryotherapy use the same word yet mean different things. *In this book, to keep the conversation simple, we will use the word "cryotherapy" or the most common abbreviation "WBC" as shorthand for whole body cryotherapy deploying only extremely cold air.*

The knowledge of cold benefits has been accumulating for more than 5000 years — the oldest medical text that refers to use of cold as a therapy was written in about 3500 BC. Medical schools in ancient Greece, Persia, and Rome all propagated cold remedies for treating a range of diseases and conditions, including relief of physical suffering, and the process was well described by the father of medicine Hippocrates as early as 400 BC. It is interesting that he also understood and insisted that wounds, exposed nerves, and acral areas (hands, feet) had to be insulated from cold rather than subjected to it; so, cryotherapy safety requirements that we use today were formulated almost 2500 years ago.

By the mid-1600s, people suffering from arthritis were commonly advised to treat the affected joints with very cold water.

In the 1800s, applications expanded. Cold was used as an anesthetic to facilitate amputations during the Napoleonic era. In 1845, James Arnott, the father of modern cryosurgery, deployed cold therapy to freeze breast, skin, and cervical tumors. A few years later, he also launched a device to combat acne and neuralgia. Unfortunately, the apparatus was not able to get cold enough for his intentions.

In other words, already in the nineteenth century it was apparent that it was not just any cold that helped but a specific type of cold, and people observed that the temperature of cold application was a significant "make or break" factor. For example, Bavarian priest Sebastian Kneipp, who wrote intensively about hydrotherapy, suggested that shorter and colder baths worked better than longer and milder, and there was a need to expose to the cold as many thermoreceptors as possible. It was his observation that the cold stimulus acts more intensely on the sensitive nerve endings in the skin if the cold water covers the whole body surface in large quantities.

The breakthrough — colder than ice

No matter how many therapeutic applications of cold were discovered, until the late nineteenth century they all involved water, snow, or ice, used either locally or as baths to immerse the entire body. The lowest temperatures available were determined by what could be achieved naturally.

The concept could only evolve when humans learned how to liquify gases. In 1898, James Dewar liquified hydrogen, reaching temperatures just 13 degrees above absolute zero. The new methods enabled the first cryosurgeries in the late 1800s and early 1900s. Then in the mid-twentieth century came the first freezers, opening the door to many more uses of cold at very low temperatures.

The first attempts to apply extreme cold to the entire human body date back to the late 1970s and early 1980s when Dr Yamauchi of Japan discovered the effects of it on his rheumatoid arthritis patients and created the first cold air therapy chamber, triggering further developments towards modern-day cryotherapy. His team's arthritis-related findings were first published in 1981 and sparked interest in medical professionals in other parts of the world.

The first cryochamber outside Japan was commissioned by German professor Reinhard Fricke in 1984. With his analysis of 40 to 60 rheumatoid patients per day, research on the mechanism of action of extreme whole-body cold and its clinical relevance had begun.

The "ice bath on steroids" misconception
that messes up the conversation

Before moving on to the details of what happens to the human body in response to being exposed to temperatures below the lowest ever registered on Earth, we need to address one common misconception that often completely messes up the conversation about whole body cryotherapy – that extremely cold air therapy is an "ice bath on steroids."

First, it does not feel similar. Those who avoid trying modern whole body cryotherapy because they "hate cold" and cannot imagine themselves entering a –100° Celsius / –148° Fahrenheit chamber if even a cold shower seems unbearable have wrong expectations. A fun fact is that just moderately cold water causes significantly more discomfort than freezing cold air because the heat transfer coefficient of water is 23.5 times higher than that of air. The difference is even bigger if ice is involved.

More importantly, it does not create the same bodily reactions. In some ways, the processes in response to cold air exposure are the opposite of those triggered by cold water immersion. Let us explain.

The human body is designed to take care of itself and is the best healer, provided that the respective built-in protective mechanisms get initiated.

The body's reaction to extreme cold is radically different from its reaction to "normal cold," such as being submerged even in ice-cold water, which is part of the environment around us in many places on Earth. The key to this difference is the speed at which the skin surface temperature drops.

Skin cooling in a chilly bath, typically between 5° and 15°C / 41° and 59°F cold, is less pronounced. The body initially keeps sending blood to the peripherals to fight the discomfort of cold water touching the skin. At the same time, heat loss due to its high transfer rate is fast. As the exposure continues, the cold starts penetrating the tissue, making the body struggle with actual, unrelenting physical cold. In 10 or more minutes, which, as studies demonstrate, is the minimum time required to achieve therapeutic benefits from cold-water immersion, the cold starts "lurking" deeper and deeper into the body, towards its core. It reaches the muscles, blood circulation in them slows, and it becomes more difficult to move. Despite the recovery benefits that this deep cooling brings, extending the time of cold exposure beyond this point can be dangerous, as it may result in hypothermia.

By contrast, skin temperature in the −100°C / −148°F environment drops by 15 or more degrees C / 27 or more degrees F in just a couple of minutes. The extreme temperatures in a cryochamber create a perceived threat to survival, not just discomfort, and the rapid cooling of the skin makes the brain initiate a process of reversing the blood flow towards the core. Preventing the core temperature from dropping is always the body's highest priority. We will explain the mechanism in more detail in the next section. For now, let us just note that, while it is freezing cold inside a cryochamber and the skin may start tingling towards the end of the session, the body engages all its heat generation capabilities, metabolism increases, blood circulation improves, and "surviving" the 3 minutes of chill is not so difficult.

The above explains why cryotherapy using extremely cold air is not "a glorified ice bath." It is not a replacement for cold water immersion, either. The two may have similar applications but have different benefits and can happily coexist. And, while people such as "The Iceman" Wim Hof keep cold bathing and winter swimming "hot," the number of cryotherapy lovers is also rapidly increasing. Cryochambers have become widely commercially available and have made cold exposures briefer, more easily attainable, and more fun.

Why all cold is not created equal and
how to choose the right type

Describing the differences between cold air therapy and an ice bath, we already gave an insight into the different mechanisms initiated in the body depending on the medium and the severity of the involved temperatures. Now, it is time to set the right expectations and help you choose the type of cold that is most likely to deliver the desired results depending on the situation.

Based on the work of Japanese and European scientists, we have now learned that the benefits of cold for pain and other unwanted symptoms are proportionate to the temperature reduction achieved and reported to the brain by the skin's thermoreceptors. It has been proven that the ambient temperature, the speed of cooling, and the level of exposure all matter. In other words, all cold is not created equal.

The benefits of whole body cold are rooted in the mechanism of thermoregulation — the body's ability to keep its core temperature within certain boundaries, despite the changes in the surrounding temperatures that affect the skin. Our nervous system constantly evaluates the environment around us and initiates processes to offset its impacts and adapt.

When the ambient environment is cold, peripheral blood vessels constrict to preserve the body's heat. The greater the difference between the skin and the outside temperatures in touch with it and the number of exposed receptors, the more pronounced the reaction and the faster the skin temperature drops to protect the core. In addition, the body seeks ways to stay warm. Among them is burning brown fat for heat, as well as making the skeletal muscles shiver.

How cold is cold enough, you may ask?

Well, it depends on the purpose.

When it comes to the reaction of the body to cold, perception of danger has proven to be the determining factor. The more extreme the environment, the sooner the body realizes that it might be in jeopardy and ensures that the organs that are most important for survival are getting enough blood to keep it going in these altered conditions. It is the rapid skin temperature drop that establishes the severity of the response – the faster the cooling, the more pronounced and systemic it is, and the more benefits can be expected.

For health improvement, not just a physical challenge and adrenaline rush, the best bet will always be colder for shorter rather than less cold for longer. It means that standing in a whole body cryochamber filled with air at –100°C / –148°F for 3 minutes will trigger a more pronounced protective reaction than sitting in cold water between 5° and 15°C / 41° and 59° F for a minimum of three times as long, while the feeling will be more extreme in the latter.

A generally healthy person looking into building the physical and psychological resilience of Wim Hof could turn to cold water to strengthen the immune system and improve the ability to cope with stress. Just know that a quick cold plunge only involves topical cooling. It does cause brief vasoconstriction but does *not* trigger the beneficial mechanisms associated with protecting the core. For that, the cold would have to be endured for much longer.

A typical cold water immersion for therapeutic purposes lasts for 10 to 20 minutes, as demonstrated by a research project carried out between the University of Miami School of Medicine and the Thrombosis Research Institute for the British Heart Foundation. During their study, patients were required to gradually extend their cold baths from 5 to 20 minutes over a 12-week period. It was only then that, in 100% of cases, the blood pressure, pulse, and cholesterol went down, oxygen capacity in the blood increased, and white blood cell count went up. Weight loss was also registered.

If the goal is performance boost, speedier recovery, or chronic pain relief, there may be a faster and less painful way. Instead of enduring regular ice baths for at least 10 minutes per procedure for several straight months, whole body cryotherapy could be not only an equal but an even better solution worth trying.

What makes modern-day whole body cryotherapy special

We all know of cases where people have endured truly extreme conditions, being buried under snow, or injured high in the mountains. Against all odds, they have been found alive, although some may have lost a limb due to freezing. Amazing, isn't it? It could only happen because in such circumstances, instead of sending warm blood to the extremities, the body does just the opposite — withdraws it from the peripheral areas to maintain the core temperature intact (crucial for survival) and to prevent hypothermia.

This same reaction results in a better blood supply to the internal organs and support of all vital functions also in a cryochamber, but the treatment time is too short to harm the vasoconstricted peripheral tissue. Just a couple of minutes later, once the cryo session is over and the threat of freezing is gone, blood gets flushed back to all corners of the body. Enhanced blood flow results in feeling warm and energized, and the body celebrates escaping the perceived danger by releasing happiness hormones — endorphins and serotonin.

Since many users of cryotherapy are involved in sports and physical performance, it is important to also mention that the cryochamber does not impact the user's mobility, which gives it a considerable advantage over cold water immersion, except for muscle recovery. During the 10 to 20 minutes of typical ice bathing, the cold penetrates quite deeply, and the muscles temporarily lose capacity. As muscle tissue needs time to return to normal, the body must rest after an ice bath; so, regardless of the time of day of this cold treatment, the athlete cannot get back to practice for hours. In contrast, the extreme cold in the cryochamber does not affect muscle tissue temperature; it only cools the very surface of the skin. Since the drop in the skin temperature is rapid, it creates a powerful illusion that the body is freezing and triggers the discussed earlier rapid response, but only minutes after exiting the extremely cold environment an athlete can continue to work out or perform.

While cold water immersion has been used for much longer, and may be more easily accessible, as well as cheaper, whole body cryotherapy chambers are becoming the go-to solution around the world, as they allow for shorter exposure, staying dry, and a much more comfortable experience overall. Also, they have a broader range of applications — not only athletic performance and recovery, but also medical purposes, vitality, and beauty. For appearance, some other forms of extreme cold therapy have also been gaining popularity in the last decade, including cryotherapy facials and body contouring relying on cryolipolysis — the destruction of subcutaneous fat cells by lowering their temperature.

There is no doubt that cold in any of its forms can deliver certain performance, health, and wellness benefits, but only one of them has a massive systemic impact on the body — whole body cryotherapy using extremely cold air. So, let us narrow the conversation down to only this most impactful aspect of the many "faces" of cold, the incredible versatility of which the wellness world has just started discovering.

In this type of application, depending on the equipment in use, the treatment temperatures fall below –85°C / –121°F and the exposure of the entire body lasts for up to 5 minutes with the purpose of tricking the brain into thinking that survival is in jeopardy and making it initiate the most powerful protective mechanisms. What it means will be discussed in the following chapter.

***

Chapter summary

Humans have been using cold water and ice for therapeutic purposes for at least 5000 years. Rooted in ancient Greek, the word "cryotherapy," which translates as "cold cure," has emerged as an umbrella term to include all applications of low temperatures. Modern-day cryotherapy, involving extremely cold air and exposing the entire body to it at once, was born in Japan in the late 1970s as a method to relieve rheumatoid arthritis pain. More and more uses and benefits have been discovered since its adaptation in Europe in the 1990s, and the therapy has seen a massive growth in popularity after entering the US market in 2010.

Whole body cryotherapy, despite being referred to as "a glorified ice bath," is more powerful and versatile than cold water immersion or any other application of cold. It has been established that shorter and colder sessions are more effective than longer exposures to milder temperatures. Rapid cooling of the skin surface leads to a massive thermoregulatory response that has benefits for performance and recovery, pain of various kinds, physical and mental health, appearance, and longevity.

Chapter 2

What Whole Body Cold Does to the Body

By consciously stressing the body physically, physiologically & psychologically, we exercise our adaptive mechanisms. So, when any type of stress comes to us out of our control, we're much better equipped to handle it.

— The Iceman Wim Hof

The most significant contribution to our well-being that we can ever make is proactively investing in our health. Sure, we need to nurture other segments of life, but if any function of the physical body is impaired, the ability to enjoy the return on other investments such as career, business, relationships, or anything material may be in jeopardy.

Life has a lot to offer, and no one wants to be unable to experience the happy moments in life because of chronic pain, illness, or disability. Not now, not ever, regardless of age! We all share this understanding yet find it difficult to let go of harmful lifestyle choices. It takes effort.

Although holistic wellness practices such as cryotherapy cannot replace the need for good nutrition, exercise, sleep, or practicing mindfulness, they can support all our other efforts and help us experience positive change faster. Even one brief session of whole body cryotherapy may cause a rapid influx of energy, boost mood, improve motivation, relieve muscle or joint pain, and lead to a night of sleeping like a baby.

How can a brief exposure to extreme cold do that? Let us explore the mechanisms behind these improvements and explain the cascade of reactions that whole body cold initiates.

The body's embedded mechanisms for self-healing and self-regeneration

The human organism is a complex self-regulating system that is designed to adjust to changes in the external environment to maintain optimal functioning.

Steady core temperature, also known as body temperature, is the most important aspect that needs to always stay within safe limits. It must be kept within a narrow range, between 36.2° and 37.7°C / 97.2° and 99.9°F, and our thermoregulatory system takes care of this. The balance the body continuously maintains between the external and internal environments is referred to as homeostasis.

The thermoregulatory system consists of:

- The peripheral thermoreceptors — specialized nerve cells found throughout the skin, able to detect and signal environment temperature changes. Their concentration is higher in the upper body, and, interestingly, the number of cold receptors is more than three times the number of nerve endings registering heat.
- The central thermoreceptors in the hypothalamus — a small area in the brain which acts as a thermoregulation control center.
- The effectors, including peripheral blood vessels, skeletal muscles, and sweat glands.

Any discrepancy between the temperature information from the peripheral receptors and the target temperature causes stimulation of either heat production or heat dissipation. In the case of exposure to low temperatures, the body reacts by turning up heat production, achieved through constriction of cutaneous blood vessels, which draws the blood towards the core to keep its temperature steady and increases blood pressure

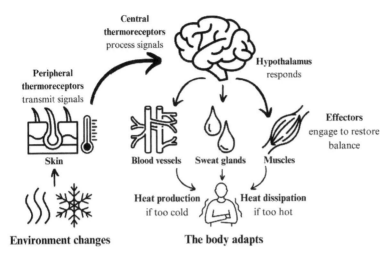

Central thermoreceptors process signals

Hypothalamus responds

Peripheral thermoreceptors transmit signals

Effectors engage to restore balance

Skin

Blood vessels   Sweat glands   Muscles

Heat production if too cold   Heat dissipation if too hot

Environment changes   The body adapts

The Elements of the Thermoregulatory System

and accelerated metabolism to produce heat by burning brown fat, also called non-shivering thermogenesis. In some cases, shivering of the skeletal muscles also gets engaged. This is a normal, healthy reaction, although comparatively rare.

The described self-regulatory mechanisms of the body, though embedded, can be compromised by many factors, including stress, injury, illness, choice of diet, and lifestyle. As a result, the body stops working to its best ability. This is where external stimuli such as whole body cryotherapy can help.

WBC uses brief thermal shock, which has proven to be one of the most effective ways to wake up the body's natural capacity for self-healing, self-recovery, and self-rejuvenation. The extremely cold, not just cold environment is important, because the body is smart and always strives to conserve energy. Only those temperatures perceived as a threat to survival cause the brain to immediately prioritize staying alive over any other task and engage the powerful protective physiological reactions that the body is capable of and that we are seeking. The cold is just a trigger in this process.

What happens when bare skin meets
extreme temperatures

To explain the truly massive response of the body to just 3 minutes of cold during a whole body cryotherapy session, we must refer to the mechanism of fight-or-flight. Let us take a minute to dissect the processes that the body undergoes during and just after the extreme cold exposure, as it is crucial to understanding the numerous advantages that whole body cryotherapy has over any other holistic wellness treatment, making it, possibly, the world's best-kept secret against inflammation and pain, among other benefits that we will explain a bit later.

The fight-or-flight response, also called the acute stress response, is a powerful and complex physiological reaction that plays a critical role in how we deal with physical stress in our environment. The term represents the choices that our ancient ancestors had when faced with danger. They could either fight or flee. Regardless, the body is prepared to trigger physiological and psychological changes necessary to avoid potential injury or death. They are involuntary, since excluding any hesitation that might delay the reaction is crucial for success.

The stress response to the nonsurvivable cold used in WBC begins in the brain as soon as it receives signals from the skin about the ambient temperature change. When the amygdala, the "fear center" of the body, perceives danger, it instantly sends a distress signal to the hypothalamus — the brain's "command center" which controls such involuntary bodily functions as breathing, blood pressure, heartbeat, and the dilation or constriction of key blood vessels and small airways in the lungs, called bronchioles. The hypothalamus communicates with the rest of the body through the autonomic nervous system and ensures that we have the energy to fight or flee.

It is important to understand that the same responses get triggered by both real and imaginary threats. In whole body cryotherapy, there is no fear other than that coming from the cold receptors in the skin, which are signalling that the body is surrounded by extreme temperatures. Because we know what to expect, the mind stays calm, and only the physical reactions that we cannot consciously control take place, enabling us to reap the full range of benefits.

The autonomic nervous system has two components — the sympathetic and the parasympathetic. One ensures alertness; the other brings calm. The sympathetic nervous system gets engaged first and acts like a gas pedal in a car. Its fight-or-flight response provides the body with a burst of energy so that it can respond to the perceived danger of WBC.

How exactly does it work? In response to the alarm that it's too cold to survive, the hypothalamus sends signals through the spinal nerves to the adrenal glands. These glands respond by pumping the hormone epinephrine (also known as adrenaline) into the bloodstream. This brings on several physiological changes. The heart beats faster than normal, pushing blood to the muscles, heart, and other vital organs. Pulse rate and blood pressure go up. Small airways in the lungs open wide. This way, the lungs can take in as much oxygen as possible with each breath. Extra oxygen is sent to the brain, increasing alertness.

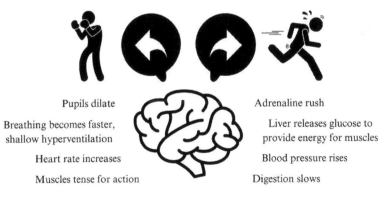

Pupils dilate

Breathing becomes faster, shallow hyperventilation

Heart rate increases

Muscles tense for action

Adrenaline rush

Liver releases glucose to provide energy for muscles

Blood pressure rises

Digestion slows

Noticeable effects   FIGHT or FLEE?   Hidden reactions

The Fight-or-Flight Response

Sight, hearing, and other senses become sharper. Meanwhile, epinephrine triggers the release of blood sugar (glucose) and fats from temporary storage sites in the body. These nutrients flood into the bloodstream, supplying energy to all parts of the body.

All of these changes happen so quickly that people aren't aware of them. In fact, the wiring is so efficient that the amygdala and hypothalamus start this cascade even before the brain's visual centers have had a chance to fully process what is happening.

Once the cold exposure is over, the parasympathetic nervous system gets engaged. It acts like a brake and promotes the "rest and digest" response that calms the body down after the danger has passed.

As we understand these natural reactions of the body and prime it for action by using the right triggers, we can become better prepared to perform under pressure. Even if we put all other benefits of cryotherapy aside, purposefully initiating the fight-or-flight response is a good way to prepare the body for handling all kinds of stressful situations.

But there is more!

A whole body cryotherapy session not only acts as a wakeup call for the organs and systems to perform better; like regular exercise, it also enables us to reach a higher state of physical and mental performance and overall well-being over time, relying on the principle known as stimuli–reaction–adaptation.

We will leave a more detailed explanation of this phenomenon to the next chapter but briefly touch upon the main elements here, since they will help us better understand not only the above-mentioned process which we undergo during a cryo exposure but also what happens in the few hours post-session.

So, first, there is the stimulus: it's too cold!

As mentioned before, the low temperatures of a whole body cryotherapy treatment stimulate the thermoreceptors in the skin and the signal goes to the brain.

Immediately, the brain reacts by sounding an alarm: danger!

The temperature of the air that the peripheral thermoreceptors register is perceived as a threat and the body mobilizes to withstand it.

The adaptation that follows is aimed at protecting the body temperature from falling.

The hypothalamus makes the peripheral tissue and abdominal organs constrict to avoid unnecessary heat wasting. At the same time, dilation of blood vessels happens in heat-generating organs.

During the treatment, while skin temperature is dropping, blood gets drawn into the core to keep it warm. Systolic blood pressure increases. All internal organs receive nutrients and oxygen delivered by the enhanced blood flow.

Upon exiting the cryochamber, the person experiences restoration.

Once the perceived danger is over, the blood vessels in the skin dilate and the blood rushes back to the peripheral tissues, resulting in a burst of physiological processes that were set off due to the cold exposure. The body feels energized.

Finally, recovery from the shock comes with relaxation.

As there is no more stress, "feel-good hormones" (endorphins) get released, resulting in a sense of happiness and vitality.

The benefits of this cascade of reactions include pain relief (reduced pain sensitivity), anti-inflammatory response, metabolism boost, elimination of toxins and waste products, improvement in joint function, and many others.

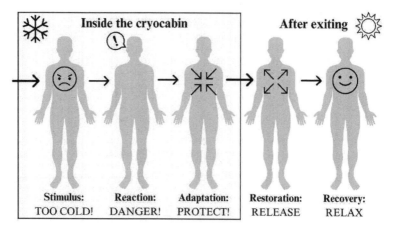

The Main Stages of the Response to WBC

The benefits build over time

As no major change happens instantly, we must distinguish between immediate, short-term, and cumulative benefits of whole body cryotherapy.

Immediately after the cold exposure, due to the dilation of peripheral blood vessels, there is enhanced blood flow to the skin and the muscles.

The relief the body feels because of having escaped from an environment that was perceived as threatening is huge — endorphins are released into the bloodstream and cause an instant feeling of being revitalized and energetic. Sudden pain relief is also often observed.

Short-term effects include reduction in pain sensitivity and improvement in mobility, metabolic efflux, reduced soreness, blunted pro-inflammatory processes, as well as feeling more relaxed, happy, and energetic. This lift lasts for several hours following a single exposure, peaking around 50 to 60 minutes after the session.

At the same time, cumulative and lasting results can only be achieved by repetitive treatments; so, for all purposes other than

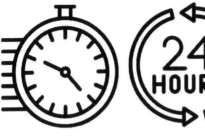
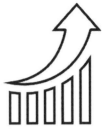

Immediate	Short-term	Cumulative
• Acute pain relief	• Lower pain sensitivity	• Chronic pain relief
• Mood lift	• Higher metabolism	• Less inflammation
• Energy boost	• Better endurance	• Building resilience

The Three Levels of Cryotherapy Benefits

immediate pain relief and boost in mood and energy, multiple visits need to be planned. As with diet and exercise, whole body cryotherapy effects become apparent and sustainable over time, usually after at least 1 month of commitment to regular treatments.

Commitment to whole body cryotherapy comes with rewards

If incorporated into a person's lifestyle and practiced regularly, whole body cryotherapy influences both the mind and body and improves general well-being, including:

- Pain relief that has a far-reaching impact on overall functioning of the body and quality of life
- Mental energy and focus that contributes to better performance at work and beyond
- Physical energy and performance, related to blood-flow stimulation and oxygenation of organs, including muscles
- Faster recovery, promoted by reduction in inflammation and pain

- Sleep, thanks to parasympathetic activation and better regulation of the circadian rhythm
- Mood and ability to combat stress, anxiety, and depression, due to pronounced hormonal responses, including the release of endorphins, serotonin, and norepinephrine and suppression of the stress hormone cortisol
- Appearance, directly dependent on skin health, tone, and texture.

Thanks to all these benefits and the little time required, just a few minutes per session, cryotherapy has become popular not only among people seeking health improvements and relief of the unwanted symptoms of various medical conditions, but also with athletes, public figures, and entertainers who have turned to cold for better performance, appearance, and longevity. In other words, there is no need to be sick, sleepless, depressed, or in pain to embrace whole body cold. It can be a major contributor to wellness in most people, regardless of sex, age, state of health, or level of physical fitness.

***

Chapter summary
The human body is a complex self-regulatory system designed to maintain stable temperature in order to support optimal functioning of all organs and systems, but numerous factors including chronic stress, injury, and illness can impair this ability. Exposure of the body to extreme cold acts as a stimulus to maintain or restore it.

The response to below-Arctic temperatures is the involuntary fight-or-flight response that activates the most powerful protective mechanisms at the body's disposal. Cold exposure triggers a danger alarm in the brain, and the adaptation includes improved blood supply to the core, engaging energy reserves, and blunting pain signal transmission, among other things. Post-treatment stages include restoration and relaxation.

Whole body cryotherapy has immediate, short-term, and cumulative benefits. Achieving the latter is only possible with commitment to at least 1 month of regular sessions.

Chapter 3

The One Thing That Changes Everything and Why Just Trying WBC Cannot Be Enough

At just 19 years old, Simeon joined the US Army after graduating from the Ranger School, one of the toughest training courses for which a soldier can volunteer. Rangers engage in close combat and direct fire battles. During the years of service, he sustained multiple injuries over his entire body that led to a post-retirement life full of pain. Being just a middle-aged man, Simeon characterized his situation as one of "lost hope" and "broken me." He was being prescribed increasingly high doses of morphine and oxycodone, was constantly sleep deprived and depressed, and was overweight. By the time he first contacted Dr Watson at Active Health & Wellness / Boise Cryotherapy, he had also developed celiac disease and was experiencing erectile dysfunction.

Just 3 days after being recommended a combination of techniques including chiropractic care, whole body cryotherapy, pulse electromagnetic field, oxygen therapy, and better nutrition, Simeon had a "crash" — he slept for 14 straight hours. In 3 weeks, he was completely off pain medications. In 2 months, the proper diet and supplements had also led to a 20-pound weight loss. No matter what the diagnosis, almost everybody possesses the ability to heal in the correct environment and by giving the body what it needs.

— Credits to Jason Watson, DC, the owner of Active Health & Wellness in Boise, Idaho, and one of the early adaptors of whole body cryotherapy in the USA

As discussed earlier, the immediate effects of cold on pain have been known for millennia, but it was discovered only recently, through studies of cold-water immersion and modern-day whole body cryotherapy involving extremely low temperatures, that series or cycles of cold treatments could lead to a gradual reduction in overall pain levels and relief of not only acute but also chronic conditions that might last for months. Numerous cases of completely discontinuing pain medication after even extended periods of depending on it have been reported in people who have been consistent and committed to frequent cold exposures. So, cryotherapy has the potential to be much more than a quick fix. It can be part of a strategy not only to improve but also to prevent health problems from developing and to maintain a good quality of life at any age.

What makes this possible?

When talking about pain reduction thanks to whole body cryotherapy, we must distinguish between three important mechanisms that enable the relief.

First is a reduction in nerve conduction velocity, or the speed at which electrochemical impulses propagate down neural pathways, meaning that transmission of pain signals during the cryo session slows down.

The second is a release of endorphins immediately following the cold exposure. These chemicals, secreted within the brain and nervous system, are known as "happiness hormones" because they activate the body's opiate receptors and diminish the perception of pain.

These two factors explain the immediate effects of cold on pain, the application that is mentioned most often.

However, the third mechanism has an even more important impact — it offsets inflammation, which is the root cause of most pain. Blood tests have demonstrated a simultaneous reduction in pro-inflammatory markers and an increase in anti-inflammatory proteins made by the immune system following a session of cryostimulation. If it is repeated often enough, the inflammation reduction becomes sustainable, enabling lasting relief.

This one reaction to cold changes everything and makes whole body cryotherapy one of the most powerful tools to battle not only the chronic pain that disturbs 1 in 5 adults on a global scale but also numerous health disorders that are caused or fueled by inflammation, which is often referred to as the cancer of the twenty-first century. As Harvard Health Publishing points out:

> Research on inflammation has created a shift in medical thinking. For two millennia it has been viewed mainly as a necessary, even beneficial, response to illness or injury. But now both observational studies and laboratory research are indicating that inflammation can be more of a bane than boon, the common, causative factor in many diseases.

As opposed to acute inflammation, which is a short-term reaction to an injury or a foreign invader in the body and a "good guy" to embrace, chronic inflammation is a long-term reaction that can result from:

- The body's failure to eliminate whatever was causing the acute inflammation, often because it is constantly fueled by poor diet and lifestyle choices and ongoing stress
- Persistent exposure to low levels of an irritant, such as pollution or pro-inflammatory foods, over a long period of time
- An autoimmune disorder that attacks normal healthy tissue, mistaking it for a pathogen that causes disease
- Obesity.

The list of conditions that involve chronic inflammation is long, from many forms of arthritis to heart disease, atherosclerosis, sciatica, ankylosing spondylitis, asthma, diabetes, ulcerative colitis, Crohn's disease, and many more, even some cancers.

Pain is a symptom of many of these conditions, whether it is muscle and joint pain, or chest pain, back pain, neck pain, or headaches. To lessen the pain, the underlying inflammation needs to be managed, including both elimination of the trigger (such as exposure to harmful chemicals, lack of physical activity, consuming inflammatory foods, stress) and introduction of anti-inflammatory treatments and habits. Many pain medications only mask the symptoms without addressing the cause. This way, the problem keeps deepening and the dose of painkillers required to handle the pain increases. Whole body cryotherapy, on the contrary, is a powerful natural way to impact the root of the problem.

But the effects of cryo go well beyond pain. It is now known that low-level untreated inflammation in the body is also a major cause of accelerated biological aging and the development of age-associated diseases. In his research publications, Dr Claudio Franceschi has even introduced a specific term — *inflammaging*. Since the year 2000 when it was first mentioned, the term has been increasingly adopted by the scientific community, and the relationship between inflammation and aging has been intensively studied.

So, to summarize, reducing the rate of inflammation in our bodies is the best defense against illness and aging. Because of the reported damage caused by long-term dependence on many medications, including seemingly harmless over-the-counter pain relievers, people have started turning to natural remedies and preventative holistic wellness practices, and brief exposures to extreme cold have been growing in popularity. Rightfully so, because whole body cryotherapy is possibly the most powerful way to fight inflammation and pain. In addition, its systemic effects on the body result in extra benefits.

Necessary prerequisites to experiencing noticeable results are commitment and following a proper protocol, though. This applies to diet, exercise, and everything else in the wellness realm. Showing up regularly will likely drive lasting improvements, while occasional and random visits will not make much difference.

**

Chapter summary

Cryotherapy has the potential to be much more than a quick pain-reducing fix. Three mechanisms are involved. Cold-induced change in the speed at which nerves transmit pain signals, and endorphin release immediately post-session often provide immediate relief. But the proven effects of whole body cryotherapy on inflammation, which causes most types of pain, may help people live a pain-free life in even quite severe cases, if only they commit to regular treatments and follow a proper protocol.

Chapter 4

What Research Says About Whole Body Cryotherapy and What's Still Missing

Cryotherapy has a long tradition in physical medicine, which is also reflected in the medicinal product guidelines of some countries. It is one of the classic stimulation therapies with the aim of restoring a misguided homeostasis.

The field of application of cryotherapy includes sports medicine, especially acute and chronic injuries resulting from intensive physical exertion. At the same time, there is a strong anti-inflammatory effect, so that acute and chronic inflammatory diseases count as indications. Polyarthritis, fibromyalgia, rheumatoid diseases, and eczematous skin diseases all respond well to whole body cryotherapy, but also neurological and neurodegenerative diseases such as spastic paresis or multiple sclerosis. Effects on mood swings, anxiety disorders and panic attacks show the wide range of therapeutic possibilities of WBC.

It is also important that there are no significant risks or side effects, apart from possible acute circulatory regulation disorders.

— Prof. Dr Harald Stossier, Head Physician
of Modern Mayr Dilijan, Member of
the Board of Complementary Medicine
at the Austrian Medical Chamber

After discussing the involuntary physiological mechanisms triggered by the body's exposure to extreme cold and explaining why and how they benefit almost every organ and system, we must connect the dots and take a closer look at the available data. It is also essential to reveal why, despite its numerous stimulating, positive effects, whole body cryotherapy is considered a non-medical treatment in most countries and is not cleared by the US Federal Drug Administration (FDA) or similar regulatory bodies to treat or cure any health condition.

In the media, you will find numerous articles using this fact to present whole body cryotherapy as being of doubtful benefit or even unsafe, yet lack of medical clearance does *not* mean that WBC has somehow failed. Like most other practices utilizing the powers of nature and the embedded abilities of the human body to heal and regenerate, it was never introduced as a cure but as a great support mechanism for the body to do a better job self-regulating. So, although modern-day whole body cryotherapy was first developed by a doctor who was seeking ways to improve the well-being of his rheumatoid arthritis patients, the cold has never been a solution on its own. It is just an external factor that stimulates the body to initiate a series of internal reactions, regulated by extremely complex systems — nervous, circulatory, and endocrine, to mention just the most important ones.

Staying alive will always be the body's priority, and it is ready to fight for it. So, creating a perceived and immediate threat to survival, as we do by exposing the body to super-low temperatures, allows us to force the organism to engage every single protective mechanism that it possesses. This massive systemic reaction makes whole body cryotherapy extremely powerful, although researching the benefits is challenging because there are so many moving parts operating at once, all of them interrelated. When we look at some isolated immediate effects of whole body cryotherapy, we only see the first few dominoes in a vast chain reaction, and assessing this in its entirety is practically impossible. The same applies to other holistic wellness practices.

The objective difficulties, which also include limited access to financing, especially when it comes to researching the effects on health conditions, explain why hundreds of cryotherapy-related studies have been conducted and published since the 1990s but every one of them has been limited in scope and size, looking only at the immediate and measurable reactions to the cold. Examples include blood tests that have shown an increase in anti-inflammatory and a decrease in pro-inflammatory markers, and an impact on white blood cell count and antioxidant levels; as well as the use of semi-subjective assessment scales, such as Hamilton's depression and anxiety rating scales (HDRS and HARS) to evaluate symptoms.

Improvements in disease symptoms have often been observed and reported, but the data obtained has not allowed researchers to draw far-reaching conclusions, and most published articles end in the statement "The effect will need to be demonstrated in future studies," or similar. As a result, we must accept the complexity-related limitations and always note that cryotherapy is not a cure for any medical condition and should not be seen as a replacement for any medical treatment. Nevertheless, it may be an extremely effective adjunct strategy to prevent or slow down the development of most inflammation-fueled conditions, improve symptoms of mood disorders, and speed up recovery, provided that the person tolerates cold well and does not have health restrictions affecting their ability to apply it.

Despite the challenges, the indication list for whole body cryotherapy has been increasingly justified and expanded over the last few decades, based on accumulating theoretical knowledge of how the body operates, clinical studies, and experience. It now includes a variety of health disorders. The terminology has also been adjusted to distinguish between the treatment of healthy subjects (when we may use the word *cryostimulation*) and the treatment of patients (when *cryotherapy* is a better descriptor).

Let us review the most-researched applications and the most-improved health conditions to inform our cryotherapy-related choices.

Researched effects of cryotherapy on the symptoms of various health disorders

Claudia had been experiencing knee pain for a few years before her doctor diagnosed her with severe arthritis and cartilage wear-down. At this point, she could barely walk, and the orthopedic surgeon with whom Claudia consulted said that a total knee replacement was inevitable. But because the technology was constantly improving, she was advised to first have some cortisone injections.

Cortisone helped for a while, but then the pain returned, and Claudia learned that she had to wait for several weeks to get another shot. There was a limitation on how often it could be done. The doctor prescribed an anti-inflammatory, hoping it would get Claudia to her next shot, but it wasn't enough. The pain was excruciating.

At that time, Claudia's massage therapist, Dawn Woodring, opened Rivanna Cryotherapy Recovery Center and suggested trying whole body cryotherapy to ease the pain. Claudia committed to daily sessions, and in just 1 week her pain was almost gone. Now, as a woman in her seventies, she does cryotherapy weekly to stay pain-free. She has indefinitely postponed the knee replacement and no longer needs cortisone injections.

— Claudia's story was published in *Woman's World* on December 2, 2019. Credits to Dawn Woodring, LMT, the owner of Chill Cville in Charlottesville, Virginia

Cryotherapy for rheumatoid arthritis

The list of medical conditions for which positive effects of whole body cryotherapy have been adequately proven usually begins with arthritis and chronic pain of various kinds.

Arthritis is not a single disease but an informal way of referring to joint pain or joint disease. In fact, there are more than 100 different types of arthritis and related conditions. In one way or another, they affect 1 in every 3 to 4 adults worldwide, the most widespread diagnosis being degenerative osteoarthritis and autoimmune inflammatory rheumatoid arthritis.

Common arthritis symptoms include warming and swelling, joint pain, stiffness, decreased range of motion, and fatigue. Severe cases can result in chronic pain and inability to do daily activities. The joint damage can become permanent, and other organs can be affected over time. For example, people with rheumatoid arthritis present a cardiovascular mortality rate that is 50% higher than in healthy persons and not related to the traditional cardiovascular risk factors, such as hypertension, use of tobacco, or physical inactivity. Several studies have shown evidence that the major risk of developing cardiovascular problems in people suffering from rheumatoid arthritis is inflammation.

Thanks to the "fathers" of modern-day whole body cryotherapy, Japanese doctor Toshiro Yamauchi and German professor Reinhard Fricke, who were seeing dozens of patients suffering from rheumatic diseases 30 to 40 years ago, enough evidence of the benefits of cryotherapy has been accumulated. As a result, German Statutory Pension Insurance, for example, has listed whole body cryotherapy in its "Classification of therapies used for medical rehabilitation" with indications for "Inflammatory joint diseases and pain syndromes" to improve function and reduce inflammatory activity and pain. Similar endorsements have been made in some other European countries.

It is important to note that arthritis is a progressive illness which, despite all the advances made in its therapy to date, still counts as uncurable. The symptoms are also likely to intensify with age, but they can be mild or moderate and remain unchanged for a long period of time. In line with minimizing the symptoms, the goal of treatment, which needs to begin as soon as possible, is to halt or delay the progression of the disease. It requires action on the underlying inflammation.

"I am a strong believer in the window of opportunity, which probably spans two years after symptom onset," says Dr S. Kazi, MD, Associate Professor of Internal Medicine and Chief of Rheumatology at the Dallas VA Medical Center. "If rheumatoid arthritis goes untreated for two years, the majority of people will develop joint erosion, indicating disease progression."

Unlike local therapies, whole body cryotherapy has the advantage of simultaneously influencing all arthritic disease foci and suppressing pain and inflammation for extended periods of time. It has been demonstrated by multiple studies that cryotherapy results in a decrease in pro-inflammatory cytokines and other inflammatory immune cells and an increase in anti-inflammatory cytokines and immune cells, in addition to the analgesic properties of cold that help improve range of motion and maintain beneficial levels of physical activity, which has been identified as an important strategy for maintaining joint function and controlling inflammation naturally.

Clinical observations suggest that with the right treatment protocol, optimally five or more sessions per week for a minimum of 2 to 4 consecutive weeks, whole body cryotherapy may help achieve effects that can still show up 3 to 6 months after the completion of therapy, including:

- Improvement in general well-being
- Pain reduction

- Reduction of inflammatory signs such as swelling and warming
- Improvement in general mobility and joint function, reported by up to 60% of the participating patients
- Reduction in intake of glucocorticoids and nonsteroidal antirheumatics, observed in 35–40% of cases.

Regular maintenance visits once or twice a week in combination with diet and exercise may make the improvement permanent. Even some cases of patients going into a complete remission have been reported after committing to cryotherapy for extended periods of time as part of their lifestyle.

The evidence clearly shows that improvement is possible, but no one should rely on whole body cryotherapy alone. As arthritis is a systemic disorder that impacts the entire organism, its treatment must also be complex, from medication and, in the case of rheumatoid arthritis, antibody therapies to a proper nutritious diet that is free of pro-inflammatory foods, exercise, and psychological treatment. Whole body cryotherapy can be understood in this context as an adjuvant physical therapy, not a substitute for other proven therapies, even if it has reportedly resulted in reduction in drug consumption in a statistically significant number of cases.

Cryotherapy for ankylosing spondylitis

Just like rheumatoid arthritis, ankylosing spondylitis or AS, also known as Bekhterev's disease, is an autoimmune chronic inflammatory rheumatic disease — one of the many forms of arthritis. As opposed to rheumatoid arthritis, ankylosing spondylitis is comparatively rare. It causes swelling between the vertebrae, the disks that make up our spine, and in the joints between the spine and pelvis, resulting in pain and stiffness. Severe cases can leave the spine hunched.

While this condition may "only" affect about 1.5% of the population, that means hundreds of thousands of people in the USA alone. It also deserves attention because a predisposition to ankylosing spondylitis seems to be genetic and its development often begins in a person's teens and young adulthood. About 80% of cases present themselves before the person turns 30, and 95% by age 45.

Although there is no known cure to date, progression of ankylosing spondylitis can be slowed by keeping the back strong and inflammation low through medication, exercise, and various therapies, including WBC. Thanks to research findings, cryotherapy has now become a solid component of ankylosing spondylitis treatment and, to prevent progression of the disease, it must begin at the earliest possible stage. It just needs to be remembered that we are only talking about symptom control, and the best approach to getting the upper hand over any medical condition is always complex and must be supervised by a physician.

As far as whole body cryotherapy is concerned, the recommended protocol for ankylosing spondylitis does not differ from rheumatoid arthritis treatment. For therapeutic purposes, it is always suggested that a person should undergo cryotherapy once daily for several consecutive weeks. The longer the breaks between sessions, the longer it takes to achieve the desired progress. With consistency, one can usually achieve recession of the inflammation, relief or elimination of the pain, reduction in oxidative stress medication intake, and an improvement in joint mobility. Relief can last for up to 2 months following the course of 10 to 20 cryotherapy sessions. In some cases, improvement for half a year has been reported. The risk of developing atherosclerosis could also be effectively minimized.

To mention an example of what could be achieved, we can refer to the work of Agata Stanek and colleagues, who once compared a group of ankylosing spondylitis patients doing whole body cryotherapy followed by kinesiotherapy for 10 straight days to a group that only did kinesiotherapy. Progress assessment included two indexes: BASDAI or Bath Ankylosing Spondylitis Disease Activity Index, which is a validated diagnostic test used to determine the effectiveness of a therapy for the treatment of ankylosing spondylitis, and BASFI or Bath Ankylosing Spondylitis Functional Index — a self-administering questionnaire that evaluates, on a visual analogue scale, functional limitation in patients with ankylosing spondylitis. In the whole-body cryotherapy group, BASDAI improved by 40%, as opposed to a 15% improvement in the "kinesiotherapy only" group. BASFI changed by 30% and 16%, respectively.

Cryotherapy for multiple sclerosis

Numerous clinical observations have now been published that underline the positive effect of whole body cryotherapy also in people diagnosed with the debilitating immune-mediated chronic inflammatory disease of the central nervous system known as MS or multiple sclerosis.

In MS, the immune system attacks the protective sheath covering the nerve fibers. The resulting nerve damage disrupts communication between the brain and the body. The symptoms can include tingling or pain in different parts of the body, impaired coordination, dizziness, fatigue, slurred speech, double vision, or loss of vision. Progression of the disease may leave the person disabled.

Since disease activity and damage continues within the central nervous system even when no new symptoms are present, once MS is diagnosed a long-term disease-modifying therapy is crucial.

Although it is believed that multiple sclerosis cannot be cured, treatment can help lessen symptoms, speed up recovery from attacks, and even alter the course of the disease. The reported benefits of whole body cryotherapy include slowing of the disease progression, possibly by impacting the underlying inflammation, and relieving its symptoms, such as pain and fatigue. Data also shows that whole body cryotherapy improves the antioxidant capacity of the organism, helping reduce oxidative stress, known to cause degenerative changes in the nervous system that are often involved in MS on top of the immune-mediated dysfunction.

In several consecutive studies led by Elzbieta Miller, researchers have compared changes in the total antioxidative status and activity of chosen antioxidative enzymes in patients with MS before and after using whole body cryotherapy. The results demonstrated that 2 weeks of cryotherapy once daily resulted in a significant increase in total antioxidative status in comparison to the reference group that did not use whole body cryotherapy, so it was concluded that exposure to extremely low temperatures might be a solution when trying to suppress oxidative stress in people suffering from MS. Another study demonstrated that cooling before exercise improved multiple sclerosis patients' functional and exercise capability, as it reduced the damaging effect of post-exercise hyperthermia.

Based on the findings, whole body cryotherapy is reported to be potentially instrumental in improving the overall well-being of multiple sclerosis patients, especially in conjunction with exercise. The results start showing after ten consecutive treatments but are most sustainable after 20; however, due to the complex nature of the disease, an open, ongoing conversation between the patient and their doctor about whether and how to use whole body cryotherapy is an absolute requirement. More than in other cases, it is of key importance to determine the individually required and tolerable dose of whole-body exposure to cold, depending on the person's ability to adequately react to the extreme cold stimuli.

Cryotherapy for anxiety and depression

When it comes to the most-reported effects by those who have made whole body cryotherapy part of their lifestyle, the top three include pain relief, sleep improvement, and impact on stress and mood. The latter is attributed to activation of the parasympathetic nervous system and to the release of endorphins and serotonin post-session, as the body celebrates escaping the perceived threat to survival that WBC represents. Recent publications also show a relationship between inflammation and dopamine levels in the brain that contribute to motivational impairments, suggesting that inflammation reduction supported by whole body cryotherapy may be instrumental in reducing depression.

Based on diverse and well-founded experiences of whole body cryotherapy leading to an improvement in mood and a leveling of the state of agitation, studies have been carried out to test its potential impact on depression and anxiety.

Most of the available research to date has been performed by Joanna Rumaszewska and colleagues. As in all other cases, the sample sizes and methodology limitations do not justify drawing far-reaching general conclusions, but the observations allow us to recommend whole body cryotherapy as a symptomatic, supplementary treatment option for affective and depressive disorders.

Across the board, the registered improvements in mood following whole body cryotherapy have been statistically significant. It has been established that, considering patients' general condition and life satisfaction, reduction of symptoms by up to 50% could be achieved. In obtaining this data, HDRS or Hamilton's depression rating scale and HARS, Hamilton's anxiety rating scale, were used as the outcome measures. After 3 weeks of WBC, a decrease of at least 50% from the baseline HDRS scores was noted in 34.6% of the study group, while HARS decreased by 50% or more in 46.2% of the study group.

A better mean state was observed with respect to 11 of the 14 components of the anxiety scale (except the gastrointestinal and genitourinary symptoms) and 12 of the 16 components of the depression scale, in line with 6 components of the life satisfaction scale, such as physical well-being, physical condition, domestic activity, professional activity, personal interests, and general satisfaction in life.

In the presence of depression symptoms, improvements in sleep have been the most noticeable. The improvement rate observed was 91% for difficulty falling asleep, 98% for sleep interruptions, and even 100% for early awakening. The improvement by 80% regarding suicidal tendency also reached statistical significance. This is an important finding, since, according to the US National Institute of Mental Health, major depression is one of the most common mental disorders in the United States, and suicide is the third leading cause of death.

It has also been observed that the worse the mental state of the individual is prior to the cryotherapy, the stronger its effect. The best results have been achieved in patients with severe depressive symptoms, in women, and in people with spinal pain.

Following the science, we can suggest that the cryotherapy protocol to achieve a noticeable and lasting improvement should involve once daily or as frequent as possible cold exposures for a minimum of 2 to 4 consecutive weeks. The more pronounced the symptoms, the longer the series should be.

Cryotherapy for fibromyalgia

For the health conditions discussed above, the benefits of whole body cryotherapy have been proven to the point where recommendations to incorporate it in the treatment regimen are given by medical professionals with confidence.

In many other cases, although positive treatment results have been obtained, they show less consistency, lack statistical significance, or have not yet led to agreement on how to interpret the collected data. Fibromyalgia is one of these conditions.

Fibromyalgia is a central nervous system disorder characterized by widespread musculoskeletal pain accompanied by fatigue and issues with sleep, memory, and mood. Researchers believe that fibromyalgia affects the way the brain and spinal cord process pain signals.

Although it is a rheumatic condition and one of the many forms of arthritis (disorders that affect the joints), the nature of fibromyalgia is considerably different from, for example, rheumatoid arthritis. Despite similarities in characteristics and symptoms, fibromyalgia is not an autoimmune disorder, and it is not an inflammatory condition, either; studies have shown that inflammatory markers in fibromyalgia patients stay within normal ranges.

In many cases, whole body cryotherapy has been proven to reduce fibromyalgia symptoms such as pain, fatigue, depressive mood, and impaired sleep, yet people's tolerance to cold and therapeutic success may differ and, since fibromyalgia is a nervous system disorder, not a condition tied to blood-flow impairment or inflammation, the positive outcomes of exposing the body to extreme temperatures may be less consistent. Some symptoms may even worsen. As a result, a more individual approach to turning to whole body cryotherapy is suggested.

To illustrate this, one study by Robert Kurzeja and colleagues resulted in 53% of the participants dropping out due to ineffectiveness, panic symptoms, or adverse reactions to cold, while the other 47% all experienced a decrease in pain intensity. In other studies, clear improvements after 20 to 30 cold exposures have been observed in somewhere between 40% and 80% of cases. It has also been concluded that gymnastic exercises 1 to 3 hours after undergoing cryotherapy may add to the therapeutic success of the treatment.

In general, research results suggest that patients with fibromyalgia should at least try cryotherapy. As in other cases involving pain, provided that the body reacts well to cold and no aggravation of nerves is observed, the cryotherapy protocol to achieve a noticeable improvement should involve treatments once or even twice daily or as frequently as possible for at least 2 to 4 consecutive weeks, reaching a total of 25 to 30 cold applications. The more pronounced the symptoms, the more intense the schedule should be, and for longer. Changes in energy levels and sleep quality usually show first, as early as after the first to third session, while a decrease in pain perception manifests itself after five to seven treatments and keeps improving with regularity and consistency.

Cryotherapy for other health conditions

While primarily pain-alleviating and anti-inflammatory, whole body cryotherapy has also shown results in neuronal activation and improvement of blood circulation and metabolism in the skeletal muscles. As summarized by Prof. Dr Sc. Med. Winfried Papenfuß in his book *Power from the Cold: Whole Body Cryotherapy at −110°C. A short-lasting physical therapy with a long-lasting effect*, evidence has been obtained that it may be intervening in a regulatory manner in disrupted central activity levels and playing a certain role in modulating the vascular system and numerous hormonal feedback loops.

The list of researched conditions for which some whole body cryotherapy benefits have been observed include various aches and pains well beyond rheumatic disorders, such as central muscular spasms and impaired central activity levels, skin and sleep disorders, and even bronchial asthma and tinnitus. At the same time, consensus on application recommendations is still lacking due to either insufficient size and scope of the studies or too much variety in the outcomes. More scientific studies will need to be performed to better justify or exclude the indications for which doubts still prevail. Nevertheless, we will briefly touch upon these less definitive findings, as in some cases cryotherapy may turn out to be a game changer for people who are given little hope by conventional medicine, reminding readers again that WBC does not heal or cure. It should always be seen only as an adjunct option, the usefulness of which must be assessed in each individual case by a qualified professional.

Aches and pains of a non-rheumatic nature

Patty lived with severe pain in her lower back and neck, caused by two injuries: a ruptured cervical nerve that helps control movements of the head and neck, and damage to the lumbosacral joint.

When Patty first visited CryoFit, her pain management doctor had cut her off pain medications because the dose required to manage the pain had grown to unsafe levels. She had heard of cryotherapy and said it was her only hope left. Because of the pain, Patty could not stand straight. Brian Balli, the owner of the center, had to do her intake bent over.

The pain was debilitating, but her heart was aching, too — Patty's brother had been diagnosed with a terminal illness, but she could not go and see him, as her back was too bad to fly or spend many hours sitting in a car. She thought they would never meet again.

Intense daily whole body cryotherapy helped this elderly woman manage the pain without the medications and straighten her spine again. A few months later, she boarded a plane to see her dying brother. In 3 more months, she was able to repeat the trip and attend his memorial.

— Credits to Brian Balli, the owner
of CryoFit in Austin, Texas

The spectrum of causes underlying chronic pain is large and ranges from severe organic diseases to inadequate pain treatment and psychosocial factors. Often, several causes combine to bring about a state of chronic pain.

Chronic pain cannot be understood only as a symptom of an underlying problem, for example an inflammatory process. It can last for months or years, can become autonomous, can coincide with the formation of pain memory, and can cause additional health problems, such as disrupted sleep or depression.

Based on the evidence obtained, we can say that whole body cryotherapy may potentially help alleviate:

- Headaches and migraine
- Spinal syndromes, particularly of the cervical and lumbar vertebrae
- Osteoporosis
- Back pain without an underlying diagnosis
- Pain after operations
- Phantom and stump pain
- Strain injuries, such as a pulled back muscle.

In most cases involving pain that is not caused by unattended physical damage such us a pinched nerve, an intense 4-week whole body cryotherapy course of five treatments per week or 20 once-daily exposures results in noticeable relief, yet it may be necessary to continue regular sessions for longer.

Tendinopathies

Tendinopathies are typically promoted by chronic overburdening of the connective tissue of the tendon attachments. Conditions include tennis and golfer's elbow, inflammation of the Achilles tendon, and heel pain, to mention just a few, and they generally respond to whole body cryotherapy extremely well. Experience shows that even severe pain upon movement recedes after only 15 to 20 cryotherapy treatments. The intensity of the schedule should reflect the severity of the issue. For more local pain relief, spot cryotherapy could be added to attend to the most painful inflamed areas.

Sleep disorders

Sleep improvement is one of the most frequently reported outcomes of committing to whole body cryotherapy. To improve sleep patterns, whole body cryotherapy contributes directly, via the regulation of central activity levels, and indirectly, for example through elimination of pain.

Not every difficulty in falling or staying asleep qualifies as a disorder, though, as sleep behavior is primarily a logical result of what we do while awake. Insomnia requiring therapy can only be considered to occur when sleep is disrupted continuously at least three times per week for longer than a month. A side effect of a sleep disorder is often tiredness. When this happens, whole body cryotherapy may help restore the disrupted homeostasis in central activity levels, so that sleep becomes more restful and daytime performance improves. Considerable results can be achieved after only 1 week of cold therapy, while it is important not to rely just on the benefits of cold. The causes of sleeplessness are too complex to do so.

If pain is the underlying cause of not sleeping well, it often takes just a few cryotherapy treatments to experience relief. In this case, experts suggest planning for cryotherapy sessions in the evening hours, as well as adding localized cryotherapy to achieve deeper cooling of the painful spots. The freedom from pain then allows the individual to fall asleep rapidly and reduce or eliminate the intake of analgesic medications.

Psoriasis

Psoriasis, like rheumatoid arthritis, ankylosing spondylitis, or multiple sclerosis, is an immune-mediated inflammatory disease. In this case, auto-aggression by the immune system leads to a chronic inflammation of the skin. In healthy humans, skin renews in approximately 1 month. People suffering from psoriasis experience it every 5 to 6 days. As the normal wear-and-tear process of the skin is disrupted, scale formation results. Psoriasis can also occur simultaneously with inflammation of joints. This condition is referred to as psoriatic arthritis.

Like other autoimmune disorders, psoriasis cannot yet be cured; so, attention is always focused on symptom relief, using methods from medications and ointments to interventions in the immune system, light therapy, and now also whole body cryotherapy – 2 weeks of 25–30 treatments have produced the best results.

After only a few days of cryotherapy the scaling may become less intense and the itching recede, and the therapeutic effect following a course of WBC may last for several months. The experiences have been inconsistent, though. It appears that, of all the different forms of psoriasis, typical or conventional psoriasis responds best to cold stimulus.

Neurodermatitis

Neurodermatitis is a hyper-reactivity of the organism towards the environment that results in inflammation of the skin. The reaction can be purely extrinsic (allergic), but genetic factors may also play a determining role.

Depending on the severity of the condition, up to 30 cold exposures may be necessary. The probability of an enduring therapeutic effect increases with an increasing number of treatments, while itching usually recedes within the first few days of therapy and dermatitis regresses in about a week.

Tinnitus

Isolated case studies have suggested that whole body cryotherapy may also have positive effects on the symptoms of tinnitus — ringing in one or both ears.

In one clinical study a group of 80 tinnitus patients received whole body cryotherapy in two series with a total of ten 3-minute exposures. As a result, in 4 patients tinnitus symptoms completely disappeared. Another 47 reported reduced intensity. Only 13 patients or 16% in this group experienced no improvement. A reduction in hearing loss was also established.

Bronchial asthma

Bronchial asthma is a condition of hyper-reactivity of the bronchial system.

The observed positive impact of WBC on bronchial asthma is rooted in its broad spectrum of effects. A short-term dilation of the bronchial tubes occurs. The respiratory musculature relaxes, and the general physical capacity is improved. In addition, one can assume an inhibitory effect on chronic inflammatory processes in the bronchial mucosa. But, compared to other potential cryotherapy applications that we are discussing in this section, asthma presents a relatively high risk. Although asthmatics often describe their WBC experience as highly therapeutic, it can result in a slight narrowing of the bronchi. Due to these risks, the treatment of asthma patients should be strictly administered or overseen by a doctor. Cryotherapy should also only be allowed if the previous asthma therapy has led to a stable state and if the patient can bear both the physical and psychological burdens presented by the cold exposure. If used, the duration of cryo sessions should be gradually increased from just 1 minute to 3 minutes over a period of several days.

Infantile cerebral palsy

Infantile cerebral palsy is a chronic postural and locomotory disorder characterized by a permanently increased tension in certain muscle groups, leading to defective movement patterns. It results from damage of the central nervous system before, during, or immediately after birth.

Treatment of spastic increases in muscular tone by cold is not new. Cold water baths, followed by gymnastic exercises, were used for spastic adults as well as children long before the emergence of whole body cryotherapy equipment.

Now, WBC is often recommended approximately 30 minutes before starting a mobilization therapy to help relax the spastic musculature. The results show that in about 70% of cases behavioral improvements can be achieved and sustained for several weeks. Improved mood and sleep patterns have also been observed. In about 10% of cases, however, increased irritability and difficulty falling asleep have been reported without the above positive effects. Consequently, the treatments must always be administered with close cooperation between the cryotherapist and the patient's physician or mobility therapist.

Preventing or slowing down the progression of dementia and Alzheimer's disease

The potential impact of extreme cold exposures on cognitive decline is one of the newest fields of cryotherapy-related clinical studies. It is far too early to present any definitive conclusions, but there is reason to believe that the anti-oxidative and anti-inflammatory effects of whole body cryotherapy may help reduce the oxidative and inflammatory stress responses that take place in patients with Alzheimer's and some types of dementia, thus having a positive impact on disease progression.

To conclude this summary of the potential applications of whole body cryotherapy in the care of various health conditions, we must stress once again that despite the positive findings presented here, cryotherapy is not a medical treatment and should never be seen as the sole solution to any disorder. Besides, it can also be contraindicated when certain cardiovascular system issues, infections, or tumors are present, as well as cause unforeseen adverse reactions, especially in people with allergies and nervous system impairments. To avoid complications, no treatment advice should be given by any person lacking professional credentials without consulting a doctor and/or receiving their explicit consent.

Cryotherapy for physical performance and recovery

The final hours of preparation before competition are important for performance. Recovery, preparation, and warm up protocols are evolving continuously and include passive and active modalities often developed by "trial and error" approaches. Passive modalities, such as whole-body cryotherapy (WBC), have the potential to enhance both recovery and preparation. Whole-body cryotherapy has generally been used within a recovery setting after competition or strenuous training for athletes, and in clinical settings for the general population. However, the acute hormonal, anti-inflammatory, perceptual and psychological responses yielded by a single, or repeated, bouts of WBC indicate that this practice could enhance an athlete's competition readiness when used in the hours before competition in addition to aiding recovery in the hours after.

— Excerpt from an article by E. Partridge and colleagues, "Whole-Body Cryotherapy: Potential to Enhance Athlete Preparation for Competition?" Published in *Frontiers in Physiology* on August 6, 2019

Whole body cryotherapy applications in sports, for athletic performance and recovery, have been researched more than any other WBC indication, with publications dating back to the early 1990s. In 1997, researcher O. Knüsel concluded that "Cold applications have become the most important form of passive physical therapy in sports medicine." Importantly, it has also been concluded that whole body cryotherapy applications do not cause any alterations of the blood that might be considered unethical in competitive sports.

The body always strives to achieve a homeostatic state, but the equilibrium is dynamic. If it is challenged through external stimuli such as physical exertion or exposure to extreme cold, the mechanisms to restore the lost balance get engaged. Undergoing the phase of stressing the body in a good way, followed by recovery, on a regular basis will lead to an adaptation of the organism not to the initial state but to higher performance levels. This effect is known as "supercompensation." So, it is thanks to the above-mentioned stimuli–reaction–adaptation principle that whole body cryotherapy is able to help achieve the body's dynamic equilibrium at a higher level of performance and state of well-being.

Two distinctively different applications of cryotherapy in sports are possible — a boost in *readiness* and *recovery*, with or without injury.

> *The clinical indications for whole body cryotherapy, including postoperative states, inflammatory processes, and blunt tissue damage, have led athletes to use whole body cryotherapy for therapeutic purposes. Furthermore, it has been pondered how the regulation of central activity levels seen after whole body cryotherapy, the economization in the cardiovascular system and the muscular effects can be utilized to boost athletic performance.*
>
> — Prof. Dr Sc. Med. Winfried Papenfuß

The best cryotherapy timing, frequency, duration, and temperature in athletic performance and recovery is highly dependent on the sport, the purpose, and the person's training status.

Recovery from injury

To better understand how whole body cryotherapy can help with post-injury recovery, we must take a closer look at the involved phases.

At first, any trauma or surgical intervention results in a cellular inflammatory reaction in the affected area. Tissue integrity has been compromised and blood supply in capillaries and oxygen delivery has been disrupted. The acute inflammation, although it is a necessary enabler of healing, can also have a damaging effect — secondary hypoxic injury of tissue due to an inadequate flow of oxygen and nutrients to its cells.

The inflammation causes pain and swelling and impairs tissue metabolism, restricting muscular activity, causing defective connective tissue function and proprioception, and reducing mobility. Unless this step is properly attended to, there are risks of lasting muscular disbalances, coordination issues, tissue degradation, loss in elasticity, and pain turning chronic. Through cold applications, immediate and forward-looking, the convalescence period can be considerably shortened and the tendency of the disorder to become chronic can be prevented.

Here are just a few examples of injury-related indications of WBC in athletics, listed by Dr. W. Papenfuß in his book *Power from the Cold*:

- Bruises and effusions in the musculature with inhibition of muscular activity
- Contusions near the joints, inflammatory joint processes, and distortions with tendon overstretching
- States following injury-conditioned surgical interventions
- Muscle strains and hardening resulting from inflammation and pain
- Muscular imbalances and differences between the sides
- Reactive psychological impairments and sleep disorders.

Performance

Today, whole body cryotherapy applications in sports go well beyond injury prevention and post-injury recovery. The results of numerous scientific studies support its inclusion in performance-enhancing programs.

The influence of cold exposures on performance is multifaceted and comes from proven effects such as:

- Boosted blood delivery to muscles post-session
- Economizing effect on the cardiovascular system
- Alteration of central activity levels.

The involved mechanisms have been well explained by two leading researchers in the field, Winfried Joch and Sandra Ückert. After whole body application, the improved oxygen supply to the musculature supports aerobic energy generation, meaning that the muscle resorts to anaerobic energy generation for maintaining performance later or to a lesser extent. The findings also suggest mobilization of energy reserves with endurance athletes, as cold action leads to less energy required for cooling the body, and an energy surplus becomes available. Oxygen consumption and heart rate do not increase as much, signs of fatigue occur later, and the organism appears to work more economically. Sweating is also reduced, which not only has effects on the energy balance but also promotes perfusion of the musculature. For details, we highly recommend reading Prof. Sandra Ückert's book, *Cold Application in Training & Competition: The Influence of Temperature on Your Athletic Performance.*

WBC effects on physical parameters such as cardiovascular performance, oxidative stress, hormonal feedback loops, exercise-induced inflammatory parameters, and haemolysis have also been studied and beneficial adaptations have been registered. For example, according to Giuseppe Banfi and colleagues, whole body cryotherapy should be seen as a protective function for athletes against oxidative stress, not only a way to bounce back: "The adaptive changes in antioxidant status actually become more obvious when whole body cryoapplications precede and accompany the intense training."

In addition, blood tests performed by the same group of researchers have demonstrated that "If high physical exertion is combined with cold exposure, the concentration of pro-inflammatory leukins [signaling molecules secreted from immune cells] decreases significantly while those of the anti-inflammatory leukins increase significantly. This means that inflammation can be effectively reduced in muscles after high physical exertion where whole body cold exposure is applied. The result is a protective effect against inflammation which can reduce injury of the muscle fibers and shorten recovery times."

Some findings indicate stress adaptation. As pointed out by Alina Wozniak and colleagues, "After repeated whole body cryo applications during the course of training, the cortisol level is clearly reduced compared to a control group even three days after the cold exposure."

A representative summary of all the above and more was published by Giovanni Lombardi, Ewa Ziemann and Giuseppe Banfi in *Frontiers in Physiology* in 2017: "Whole-Body Cryotherapy in Athletes: From Therapy to Stimulation. An Updated Review of the Literature."

Post-exertion recuperation

Athletes place considerable demands on their bodies when undergoing training programs to facilitate competition performance, and fast recovery is of notable concern, encompassing the restoration of physical disturbances induced by exercise, including glycogen depletion, hyperthermia, disruption of muscle fibers, and accumulation of lactate. If the body has not been given time and support to recoup its resources, the physical stress accumulates over time and can compromise homeostasis and immune function, increasing the probability of injury, illness, and the onset of nonfunctional overreaching or overtraining.

Considering these implications, experts have turned their attention to post-exertion recovery more than ever before, and whole body cryotherapy has been found to be a powerful practice that supports faster returning to a normal state of strength, health, and mind. Studies have demonstrated that whole body cryotherapy is capable of lowering activity-induced inflammation and muscle damage or soreness and delivering recuperation faster and to a greater extent than other methods.

For example, an experiment performed by Dr Christophe Hausswirth and colleagues involved nine well-trained runners and compared the speed of regaining strength after three sessions of WBC, far infrared sauna, and passive recovery. Markers of muscle damage and perceived sensations such as pain, tiredness, and well-being were recorded before, immediately after exercise, and 1 hour, 24 hours, and 48 hours later, respectively. In all the testing sessions, a simulated 48-minute trail run induced a similar, significant amount of muscle damage. The results showed that maximal muscle strength and perceived sensations were recovered after the first whole body cryotherapy session (in 1 hour), while recovery took 24 hours with far infrared sauna and was not attained through passive recovery. Three cryotherapy sessions performed within 48 hours after the damaging run accelerated recovery from exercise-induced muscle damage faster and to a greater extent than the other two modalities.

Cryotherapy protocols in sports and fitness

When it comes to cryotherapy protocol suggestions, we must take into account that athletic performance is an extremely complex phenomenon, and nothing is equally good for everyone and everything. More than in other applications, it is essential to talk about differentiation, specialization, and individualization of approaches, based on the discipline, level of preparedness, and specific abilities of every athlete, among other factors. Significantly different recommendations should be given for building strength and endurance, preparing for competitions, and recovering from exertion during the training and active seasons. For this reason, we will abstain from providing any particular protocol suggestions in sports. It has been proven that all cold applications, also including ice baths and localized cryotherapy, can bring about improved motor performance and aid in speedier recovery, but the effects depend on appropriate administration, best left to professionals.

Cryotherapy for vitality and general well-being

The most important aspect when talking about cryostimulation for general health and well-being purposes is the systemic effect that is triggered via neuronal reflex mechanisms and elicits complex responses, affecting both the physique and the psyche and involving the central and the autonomic nervous systems, cardiovascular and respiratory systems, hormonal regulation, metabolism, immune function, as well as the skin and skeletal musculature.

Although most often presented as a tool to relieve pain, manage chronic inflammation, and assist with recovery, whole body cold can be used by anyone interested in optimizing their psycho-physical abilities — for professional or leisure reasons or just to achieve a dynamic equilibrium at a higher level of performance and better state of well-being. Once again, it is possible thanks to the above-mentioned stimuli–reaction–adaptation principle involved in the body's reaction to the extreme temperatures of modern-day cryotherapy.

The word is spreading, and the number of whole body cryotherapy evangelists is growing worldwide. The acceptance of WBC is also on a continuous rise because exposure to cold can now be accomplished in a comfortable form and environment, via brief, dry sessions in a cryochamber, rather than lengthier and more difficult-to-bear cold plunges or ice baths.

Effects of cryotherapy on stress reduction and relaxation

Initially, the studies and the related discussions concerning the effects of whole body cold applications on the central nervous system were focused almost entirely on the control of chronic inflammatory processes and the perception of pain by the brain. More recent research has proven that there is more. Whole body cryostimulation modulates activity levels in the brain and contributes towards bringing about a balanced mental state, improving sleep patterns, better stress handling, and overcoming overstrain. One of the mechanisms involved is stimulation of the vagus nerve — the longest and most complex of the 12 pairs of cranial nerves that emanate from the brain. It transmits information to and from the surface of the brain to tissues and organs in many parts of the body.

The parasympathetic side of the nervous system, in which the vagus nerve is heavily involved, decreases blood pressure and heart rate and helps with calmness, relaxation, digestion, and bladder, bowel, and sexual functions. Stimulating this extremely important nerve can result in numerous benefits for the most vital functions of the body, and, according to a 2001 study, cold exposure is one of the most effective ways to do so. It can be explained by the body's natural response to low temperatures — using breath to calm down. As the body adjusts to the cold and passes a certain time frame, 45–75 seconds on average, the sympathetic fight-or-flight activity of the nervous system decreases while the parasympathetic "rest and digest" system gets activated.

The impact of cold on cardiovascular and respiratory systems

Studies into the cardiovascular and respiratory effects of whole body cold were already instigated in the mid-1980s by Prof. Reinhard Fricke. In recent years, major efforts have been made to substantiate these findings further, and good results have been achieved by groups of Polish, German, and Italian scientists.

Short-term exposure to extreme temperatures induces a desirable thermal conditioning of the blood vessels in the skin. It is an essential prerequisite for modulating blood pressure and improving oxygen supply and uptake.

A 2021 study by Magdalena Wiecek and colleagues looked at the activity of nitric oxide synthase in men in their mid-fifties to mid-sixties. Nitric oxide helps the body dilate and constrict blood vessels and can improve blood pressure and heart health. Its production is also essential because it allows blood, oxygen, and nutrients to travel to every part of the body and helps minimize aging-related oxidative stress, endothelial dysfunction, and a reduction in the bioavailability of nitric oxide. The results of the study demonstrated that 24 whole body cryostimulation sessions performed every other day resulted in inducible nitric oxide synthase concentration increase regardless of the subject's physical activity level.

The potential positive effect of WBC on the respiratory system is rooted in a broad spectrum of reactions. To mention just a few, a short-term dilation of the bronchial tubes occurs, the respiratory musculature relaxes, and the general physical capacity of the system is improved. In addition, one can assume an inhibitory effect on chronic inflammatory processes in the bronchial mucous membrane if present.

Effects of WBC on hormone release, sleep, mood, immune function, and energy metabolism

Hormones are fundamental to the proper functioning of a human body. Released from glands in the endocrine system, they serve as messengers, controlling and coordinating activities throughout the body, telling it how to breathe and how to expend energy, and regulating processes such as blood pressure, among many others.

Initially, when undergoing whole body cryostimulation, adrenaline and noradrenaline levels in the blood increase, but the adrenaline rise is short-lived. It is just a result of the agitation associated with entering the cryochamber. The increase in serum concentration of noradrenaline, likely due to the transmitter function stimulation by the extreme environment, brings about an increase in the pain threshold and contributes to immediate pain relief.

As the parasympathetic activation takes over, a significant reduction in the stress hormones adrenocorticotropin and cortisol has been registered, positively affecting stress, sleep, and the immune system, as elevated cortisol levels interfere with it, while lowering of cortisol is beneficial. Measurements also show a cold-induced increase in the number of immune cells (leukocytes), thus improving the organism's ability to deal with foreign molecules that enter the body and infections, and strengthening innate immunity.

Furthermore, sleep improvement has been reported that usually comes from an increase in the proportion of deep sleep versus the total time spent asleep and has positive implications for the overall hormonal balance. For example, although no direct correlation between cryostimulation and an increase in the growth hormone somatotropin has been established, it is known that deep sleep has an impact on whether secretion of the growth hormone that ensures cellular renewal and health of the immune cells occurs at appropriate levels.

Finally, there is no doubt that people undergoing cryostimulation experience a following elevation in mood, probably due to the release of endorphins and serotonin associated with escaping the perceived danger of the extremely cold environment.

Another interesting aspect is the behavior of energy metabolism under whole body cold exposure. On one hand, the body needs less energy to cool itself, meaning that a greater amount of energy can be allotted towards physical performance or brain function. We have already discussed the energy economization effect when explaining the impact of WBC on athletic results. On the other hand, the oxygen radicals that are an inevitable byproduct of energy metabolism can be rendered harmless more effectively, as multiple studies have demonstrated that cooling has a modulating effect on the oxidant/antioxidant balance. The reduction in oxidative stress is important in preventing the development of many health disorders and halting their symptoms, as well as slowing down aging of the body.

General recovery

Although the recovery benefits of whole body cryotherapy are most often mentioned alongside sports performance, it can also be a great tool in the process of recovering from chronic illness, serious injury, or surgical operations. While it is strongly recommended that introduction of holistic wellness methods into the recovery process be supervised by a doctor to ensure synergies between medication, physical therapy, and any other elements of the likely complex approach, cryotherapy has proven to effectively manage pain, reduce inflammation and swelling, speed up healing, and support energy and mobility.

Explanation of the positive impact is likely rooted in the above-mentioned effects on pain signal transmission, blood circulation, inflammation, enhanced production of infection-fighting white blood cells, antioxidant levels, regulation of hormones, and sleep enhancement — all important contributors to healing and the restoration of strength. Numerous cases of people getting back on their feet faster thanks to regular cryostimulation have been reported.

The link between whole body cryotherapy and appearance

You may also have heard statements that cold is an "elixir of youth," and there is sound reasoning behind this claim, although just exposing the body to low temperatures will hardly be enough.

Skin, the body's largest organ, is a visible reflection and an important indicator of the *inner health* of the organism – primarily gut health, but also inflammation, oxidative stress, and other damaging internal factors that are known to cause skin problems, from dry skin, puffiness, and acne, to eczema and rosacea.

As whole body cryotherapy has a *systemic effect* on the body, including blood circulation and antioxidant capacity improvement, inflammation reduction, metabolism boost, forced contractions of the smooth muscles that we cannot consciously control or exercise, and even mitochondrial biogenesis, it does impact appearance in a big way and contributes to smoother, better-looking skin, even if only indirectly. All the above factors are vital for cell rejuvenation, effective detoxification, and reducing signs of aging.

How can whole body cryotherapy impact biological aging?

As life expectancy in the modern world increases by 2 years per decade, there is an increasing focus on longevity. This means not just living longer but looking and performing at one's best for as many years of life as possible. The aging population is one of today's biggest concerns, and research suggests that the main enemy of longevity is inflammation, often referred to as the cancer of the twenty-first century.

Based on the data obtained, we now know that subtle but chronic low-grade inflammation is a characteristic of increasing age and a major contributor to the progression of many age-related chronic diseases. Scientists fittingly call the process *inflammaging* — aging promoted by inflammation and oxidative stress. The term was first introduced by Claudio Franceschi in 2000.

In recent years, research has demonstrated that through the implementation of healthy lifestyle interventions and nature-based therapies such as whole body cold applications, the progression of many chronic diseases can be slowed or even reversed, especially when paired with performance support and rehabilitation exercises.

In a 2021 paper published in the *Journal of Thermal Biology*, a group of scientists led by Slawomir Kujawski indicated decreased levels of inflammatory markers particularly in the age group of 55 and older, following whole body cryotherapy. They also noticed a significant improvement in short-term memory in subjects with mild cognitive impairment, concluding that "In conditions associated with cognitive dysfunction including Alzheimer's and other forms of dementia the many properties of WBC have exciting therapeutic potential."

Another contributor to aging and to the development of various health conditions is oxidative stress, also proven to be positively influenced by exposing the body to extremely low temperatures.

It just needs to be emphasized that, although whole body cryotherapy has proven anti-inflammatory and anti-oxidative properties, making it an essential part of an anti-*inflammaging* regimen, it can only deliver significant results for vitality and well-being if combined with lifestyle choices, including but not limited to proper nutrition, hydration, supplementation, exercise, stress management, healthy food intake and sleep habits, and other methods to boost cell health, for example light therapy, also known as photobiomodulation, as a healthy body requires healthy cells.

Cryotherapy and weight loss

Of all applications of cryotherapy, weight loss is probably the most controversial; so, to begin, let's make it clear that WBC is *not* a weight-loss treatment, although it can be successfully integrated into weight-loss programs.

To understand the processes behind cold-promoted slimming, the opportunities, and the limitations, we must first talk about fat.

Human beings have white and brown adipose tissue.

The "standard" white fat stores energy in fat droplets distributed around the body. They grow when the amount of nutrition supplied exceeds the pending energy requirements of the organism and when the uptake capacity of the liver and skeletal muscle to store the extra energy as glycogen has been exhausted. Most of our fat is white fat. It plays an important role in our biology, as it not only serves as an energy buffer to get us through times when there is a deficit of fuel but also provides insulation for the internal organs. Too much of it builds up in obesity, though.

The brown fat, also known as the "good fat," stores energy in much smaller droplets than white fat and is specialized in burning them for heat. Brown fat cells are packed with iron-rich energy-generating mitochondria which give them a darker color. Low temperatures are known to activate brown fat, leading to various metabolic changes in the body — in response to cold, brown fat breaks down blood sugar (glucose) and fat molecules to help maintain body temperature, burning calories in the process. This process is called non-shivering thermogenesis and is now highly regarded as a possible treatment for obesity and some metabolic syndromes.

Some research has suggested that cold may even help generate more brown fat cells and that just 2 hours of daily exposure to temperatures as high as 19°C / 66°F may be enough to turn recruitable white fat into brown. Helpful strategies include swimming in cool water, taking cold showers or ice baths, or turning the home thermostat down a few degrees, not to mention whole body cryotherapy.

Another hypothesis is that cryostimulation, if used regularly, "teaches" mitochondria to take extra food and burn it up as heat, leading to improved calorie burn over time. It was recently supported by a group of Italian researchers — Massimo de Nardi and colleagues. They tested resting energy expenditure (REE) in both lean and obese women pre- and post-cold exposure on day one and day five of whole body cryotherapy treatment, using indirect calorimetry as a measurement method. REE pre-cryo increased from day one to day five by 8.2% or about 130 kcal/day in lean study participants and by 5.5% or about 90 kcal/day in overweight subjects, suggesting that cold-induced thermogenesis could be further explored as a strategy to elevate resting energy metabolism. In our own experience, some clients committed to frequent cryotherapy sessions have been surprised by a loss of a few pounds as a side effect, yet such an outcome should not be expected — too many factors are involved in determining it.

***

Chapter summary

The massive systemic reaction to extreme cold rooted in the body's embedded readiness to fight for survival is difficult to study. Most research only addresses the first few dominoes in a vast chain reaction; assessing this in its entirety is practically impossible.

Hence the limitations. As a result, WBC is not regarded as a medical treatment in most countries and should be seen as an effective adjunct strategy rather than the sole solution to any problem. Nevertheless, despite the challenges, the indication list of whole body cryotherapy has been increasingly expanding to include health conditions such as rheumatoid and osteoarthritis, ankylosing spondylitis, multiple sclerosis, fibromyalgia, affective and depressive disorders, insomnia, musculoskeletal pains, tendinopathies, psoriasis, and neurodermatitis, to mention just a few. It has also proven to be instrumental in post-injury and post-surgery recovery, boosting physical performance and speeding up post-exertion recuperation, and more and more evidence suggests that there are numerous benefits for vitality, longevity, and beauty. An increasing number of wellness experts regard whole body cryotherapy as a low-risk and potentially high-reward practice of hormesis (good stress) that should at least be tried, except in cases when clear contraindications have been identified.

*If you are interested in having a closer look at the topics that have been studied to determine the effects of whole body cryotherapy and reading some of the papers, please visit **reinventing.cool/proof** where the list is being regularly updated.*

Chapter 5

How Much WBC Is Enough and Can There Be Too Much?

Jacqui was diagnosed with rheumatoid arthritis when she was just 40. Although she was given the best biological medications that helped keep the rather severe symptoms under control, she did not want to live like an "old person" and was continuously searching for ways to make life easier and more fulfilling, open to trying new things.

By the time Jacqui discovered whole body cryotherapy, she had already reached her late fifties, been through knee replacement and spinal fusion, and added another serious health condition — fibromyalgia, which was causing pain all over her body; so, it felt like there was nothing to lose. A few months into regular WBC sessions, Jacqui's fibromyalgia had almost disappeared, and her rheumatoid arthritis had improved to such a degree that life could finally take on new dimensions, both physically and mentally. Now, more than a year later, she keeps coming back for more. In her own words: "I'm probably not the most obvious cryotherapy devotee, but I have become one because I can't even tell you how amazing this very simple and fast treatment has been for me. Admittedly, sometimes I arrive, and getting undressed and freezing is the very last thing I want to do, but after my magic three minutes the world is a different place, and I am truly buzzing. In fact, I am so upbeat that my husband and friends have started calling me a Duracell bunny. So, thank you, Maria and

LondonCryo team, I can honestly say that you have changed my life!"
— Credits to Maria Ensabella, the founder of
LondonCryo and co-author of this book

In the previous chapter, we covered dozens of potential uses of whole body cryotherapy, some of them well proven and broadly adopted, such as pain management or recovery from a strenuous workout, many more emerging as a powerful support to diverse healthcare and preventative care practices and longevity biohacks. Now we must address the questions of dose and frequency of extreme cold exposures to achieve the results that one is seeking. Let us first review the "general truths" of designing cryotherapy protocols that work. Then, in Chapter 6, we will discuss customization, considering not only the purpose but also individual characteristics and limitations.

To begin, we must make it clear that here we can only talk about best practices. There is *no* "one size fits all" when it comes to establishing the optimal cryotherapy treatment regimen. As with exercise, nutrition, or supplementation, the length and total number of recommended applications, their frequency, and the best timing for them depend on the condition of the individual and their goal. There is also a huge difference between what's needed in acute stages of injury or illness and what is enough for maintenance.

What to expect from a single use

As with most other therapies and wellness-improving practices, a single use, although beneficial, can only generate short-term effects. A sole whole-body cryotherapy session may ease acute pain for a short while, relieve stress or tension, lift mood, or help one relax after a long day at work or physical exertion. It could be a nice cool-down on a sweltering hot day, an influx of energy after a sleepless night, a hangover relief, or an aid to overcoming jetlag after a long-haul flight. It will also serve the purpose of trying cryotherapy for the first time, but no lasting improvement of any aspect of well-being should be expected.

What one *can* count on are the physical reactions associated with "fight or flight" — blood circulation boost, the alertness that comes with the initial adrenaline rush, followed by calmness from vagus nerve stimulation, and happiness from the release of endorphins. Cold also acts as a powerful analgesic, slowing the transmission of pain signals. All of these effects are often immediate and can last for up to several hours post-exposure. Measurements show that core temperature, although impacted ever so slightly, reaches the lowest point about 1 hour after leaving the cryochamber, indicating that the processes triggered during the cryo session take time to unfold and deliver all their benefits.

Committing to a series of sessions

"Multiple use" refers to undergoing a certain number of cryotherapy sessions within a defined timeframe. The length and intensity of the therapy should be informed by the person's reason for showing up and the gap between their current and desired states of being. Most often, such concentrated "campaigns" of treatment, obtained as packages, are related to post-injury or post-surgery recovery or improvement of the symptoms of a medical condition. The recommendation to incorporate WBC may or may not be given by a physician.

To accumulate the benefits fast and to ease the inflammation and pain involved in most such cases, regularity of cryotherapy treatments is the key success factor. Research usually supports at least 10 days and up to 4 weeks of whole body cryotherapy as often as possible – five to seven times per week or, in severe cases, even twice daily. Many studies have led to the same conclusion — that 20 or more sessions deliver the fastest and longest-lasting improvement.

Another reason for limiting the number of sessions may be availability — a comparatively short stay at the treatment place, which may be a hotel, a rehabilitation center, or a resort. Although at least five sessions are generally recommended to start feeling the impact of cryotherapy, even a few cold exposures come with certain benefits which should not be neglected.

Designing a cryotherapy routine

"Continuous use" means integrating cryotherapy into one's regular wellness regimen. Just like eating healthily or working out, whole body cryotherapy has most benefits if practiced routinely, from once or twice a week to as often as daily. For the best value for money, committed users typically opt for large packages of treatments or memberships available at most places offering cryotherapy and adjust their schedules to their status and availability. For example, more stressful times at work, studying for an exam, or preparation for a sports event such as running a marathon will likely lead to a more intense cryotherapy regimen, followed by a maintenance mode of a session every three to five days or so.

It is important to note that in sports and fitness, *timing* of treatments is often more important than frequency. For example, if athletic performance is wanted, to achieve muscle oxygenation and the energy optimization effect discussed earlier, whole body cryotherapy treatment could be planned 1 to 2 hours before the event, training, or competition. For recovery purposes, to prevent lactic acid buildup and to reduce muscle fatigue, the session should follow the event with as little delay as possible. If the treatment does not take place within the first 24 hours, it will likely produce very little effect, if any. On the day of an important event, two cryotherapy treatments may be scheduled — one for readiness and one for faster recuperation and, although common best practice is observing a break of a few hours between consecutive sessions, this rule can be broken, especially under the professional supervision of a trainer or a doctor.

Can cryotherapy be overdosed?

If WBC is practiced randomly or the total number of sessions is low, it is likely that the body will not adapt fast enough to show a noticeable difference, but can there be too much whole body cryotherapy? The short answer is "yes," it is possible.

First, the body's reaction to cold exposures becomes less amplified over time. The human organism is very adaptable and, as it gets used to the extremely cold temperatures, the shock effect lessens. Over the course of many treatments, some level of habituation is inevitable, although it is difficult to predict when it might set in and how pronounced it would be.

One way to identify the moment of when it happens is by measuring blood pressure before and after the treatment. The systolic pressure (the upper number) should go up by at least five points over the cold exposure, due to the body drawing blood to the core for its protection. If blood pressure does not change or reduces, the thermal shock mechanism is not working properly.

Does this mean that the treatments should be put on hold? It depends!

For short-term objectives such as sports recovery or acute pain relief, a strong thermal shock is wanted to stimulate peripheral blood flow and to boost the anti-inflammatory effect and release of endorphins. This implies that habituation is *not* wanted and should be prevented by either increasing the dose (the length of exposure or the speed of cooling) at every second treatment or by incorporating longer breaks between exposures to let the body reset.

For long-term objectives such as treating the symptoms of rheumatoid arthritis, chronic pain, or depression, it is not about the thermal shock but about the continuous stimulation of the thermoregulatory responses; so, treatments may be continued even if habituation is observed.

Secondly, although rarely, it is possible to experience a sudden adverse reaction to cold after five or more treatments, especially if the schedule has been intense. For example, cold panniculitis that shows as rash — red, risen skin surface in the form of plaques, papules, or nodules — is an inflammatory response of the subcutaneous fat to cold exposure, usually repeated. Side effects like these are not dangerous and do not require medical attention; they typically disappear within 2 to 3 weeks, but cryotherapy sessions during this period must be discontinued.

***

Chapter summary

The recommended dose, frequency, and timing of extreme cold exposures vary greatly depending on the person's condition, intention, and individual characteristics, but a few general rules apply. Single or random use, though beneficial, will not deliver any lasting results. Multiple treatments, usually planned to reduce the symptoms of a health condition or to support a short-term goal, deliver more noticeable improvement faster if repeated at least 20 times as often as possible, up to once or even twice daily. Continuous use of cryotherapy can be a great lifestyle adjustment, but more is not necessarily better. The body's reaction to cold is likely to get less pronounced over time. Such habituation, if not desired, can be overcome by taking occasional breaks in the treatment schedule.

Chapter 6

Creating a Customized
Roadmap of Using Cold to Reach the Goal

Tiago, a 40-year-old banker, loved running. In his early thirties, he completed the New York Marathon and continued with a half-marathon at least annually, and occasional 10K races, until it had to stop because he had developed a condition called hip impingement, meaning that the ball of the hip joint was pinching up against the cup, causing stiffness and pain. In addition, the long hours spent at the desk in front of a computer every day were resulting in severe discomfort in his back and shoulders. Osteopathy and physiotherapy sessions were delivering short-term improvements but weren't enough — the pain kept returning. Some doctors were suggesting surgery but would give no guarantee that it would cure the problem.

It was Tiago's wife Rita who suggested trying whole body cryotherapy; he hadn't even heard about it. Skeptical at first that cold would do much for the chronic hip issue, he decided to give it a shot and, in addition to exercising twice a week with a physical therapist, followed the cryocenter's recommendation to commit to daily cryotherapy for two straight weeks. As busy as he was, he managed to schedule the sessions around his professional commitments, carving out time either early in the morning, during lunchtime, or on the way home. Here is what he had to say upon completion of the 10-day streak:

"The back and shoulder pain started to improve by the second session and completely disappeared by the

fourth session. In the beginning of the second week, the pain in my hip had also improved a lot. I was not feeling it every day anymore. With the end of the sessions, I expected it to come back, but it's been five days now of no cryotherapy and I am still feeling good and pain-free. There were also a couple of things I wasn't expecting but that were a good surprise! I had more energy since the first session and noticed a general improvement in my well-being. Having 'tested' cryo in the morning, lunchtime, and at the end of the day, I can say that for me it worked best after work because I felt more relaxed and less tired when I got home. But I guess it could be different for other people."

— Credits to LondonCryo Belgravia

At this point, we have covered the physiological mechanisms triggered by whole body cryotherapy in line with their general benefits, potential applications, and limitations. We have also given an insight into what results could be expected depending on the number, frequency, and timing of extreme cold exposures. But one important element is still missing — customization of the approach, considering not only objective circumstances but also personal characteristics and expectations. The optimal cryotherapy regimen will always be different for different people and must balance the following three aspects:

- *Effectiveness* to produce the expected outcome
- *Safety* to prevent any adverse reaction or injury
- *Perception* to ensure a positive experience and tolerable conditions regardless of the individual's susceptibility to cold.

It may also have to be adjusted over time as the situation changes.

The purpose of this chapter is to discuss the factors involved and help you combine them for maximum benefit.

Planning with the result in mind

In wellness as much as in everything, the best strategy depends on the result that needs to be achieved. Paraphrasing the Cheshire Cat from *Alice in Wonderland*, which way to go depends a good deal on where you want to get to. If you don't much care where, then it doesn't matter which path to take. As highlighted earlier, the best frequency of cryotherapy sessions for general well-being purposes will be considerably different from the schedule to achieve rapid improvement in the symptoms of a health condition. Treatment timing to boost athletic performance will not be the same as for muscle recovery. The total number of cold exposures required to ease chronic pain will be much higher than it would be to improve mental clarity and concentration while preparing for an important exam. So, the first question that needs answering before embarking on the ship of cryotherapy is: *Where to?*

Common goals include pain relief, reduction in symptoms of being unwell such as fatigue, taming inflammation post-injury or surgery, handling stress, deepening sleep, boosting mood, improving skin condition and tone, and speeding up recovery after illness or physical exertion, to mention just a few. Depending on the answer, decisions need to be made with regard to the following:

- Treatment *dose.* This is established by the speed of cooling in combination with the duration of the cold application. Nitrogen-cooled cryotherapy devices allow for temperature adjustment; electric chambers rely on airflow to create a windchill effect. A typical length of one treatment falls between 2 and 4 minutes. Finding the optimal balance requires a bit of experimentation because, as will be discussed shortly, individual characteristics play a significant role, but there is also experience that can be relied on. It suggests that painful inflammatory conditions, for example, respond best to a higher dose of cold while a session in pre-competition preparation should be kept shorter and/or be milder.

- The total *number of treatments* during a serial application. We discussed the considerations and the likelihood of developing some level of habituation over time in Chapter 5. This factor is most important if improvement in symptoms of a medical condition is desired, and the suggested target in most cryotherapy-related studies is 20 or more.
- The *frequency* of exposures. Again, this matters most for pain management and health improvement. To build the momentum, the initial schedule is usually intense — one or even two sessions per day or, if that is not attainable, as often as possible. Without an urgent need or for maintenance purposes, twice weekly is usually considered the "golden middle."
- The *time of day* or *time relative to physical activity*. This is particularly important in pain management and sports performance and recovery, as well as in sleep enhancement. Arthritis or multiple sclerosis patients, for example, may cryo shortly before physical activity, as it reduces pain associated with movement, improves range of motion, and, in the case of MS, lessens the extent of post-exercise hyperthermia.

Another variable to consider is the *interval* between consecutive serial applications; this matters most when whole body cryotherapy is used to manage the symptoms of an incurable chronic medical condition. Depending on how severe the disease is, the period of relief may last anywhere between 1 and

6 months; so, the strategy could be going "all in" for a month, then taking a break or relaxing into a maintenance mode for some time, then returning to another round of more intense therapy, and so on.

Excluding health risks

Whole body cryotherapy is a safe treatment aimed at strengthening the body's embedded protective properties against environmental stressors. Adverse events appear to be rare in relation to the extent to which WBC has grown worldwide. Only isolated cases have been reported to date, usually in combination with triggers such as hormonal imbalances, drugs, or physical stress. Nevertheless, extreme cold exposure may pose health risks for people with certain medical conditions, especially those associated with poor cardiovascular health, acute respiratory problems, blood clotting, or allergies.

The person undergoing cryotherapy needs to be able to cope with blood pressure and blood flow increase during and just after the treatment. Hence absolute contraindications such as untreated high blood pressure above 160/100 mm Hg, a heart attack that occurred less than 6 months ago, congestive diseases of the cardiovascular and respiratory systems, unstable angina pectoris, a cardiac pacemaker, peripheral circulatory disorders, acute phlebitis, venous thrombosis, severe anaemia, acute kidney/urinary tract diseases, tumors, seizures, skin infections, and cold allergies. In all these cases, cryotherapy should only be administered if specifically prescribed or explicitly cleared by a doctor.

Relative contraindications that require caution and for which a person undergoing cryotherapy should be overseen by a medical professional include cardiac arrhythmias, heart valve defects, ischemic heart disease, Raynaud's syndrome, polyneuropathies, immunosuppression, vasculitis, and claustrophobia. The latter is less of a problem in the cylinder-shaped nitrogen-cooled cryotherapy devices leaving the person's head above the edge of the cold cloud and allowing for close interaction and eye contact with the operator throughout the session, but can result in a panic attack in one of the enclosed walk-in chambers, especially in high humidity environments that cause fogging.

Proper intake plays a crucial role in identifying and minimizing the risks prior to the first cryotherapy session. Not every condition has been researched, and every person has a unique set of individual characteristics, medical history, and tolerance limits. For these reasons, anybody suffering from a serious illness or feeling uncertain about a health-related condition should first turn to the attending physician to evaluate whether cryotherapy is safe to perform. To review the list of most common health concerns, visit **reinventing.cool/contraindications**.

Accounting for individual characteristics

In addition to health and physical conditions, there is another factor that plays an important role in ensuring compliance and providing whole-body cryotherapy safely, and this must not be neglected. It is the significant difference in how individuals respond to cold.

In the 1950s, it was observed that US troops of African origin stationed in Alaska experienced frostbite and other adverse reactions to cold much more often than their Caucasian peers. Researchers have since demonstrated that in the same low-temperature environment the variation in skin temperature drop between individuals can be vast. This phenomenon must be remembered when considering whole body cryotherapy.

But the influencing factors include not only the person's race. There is also age, gender, body fat and muscle mass, physical and emotional state, skin tone and skin status, and the level of fitness. For example, women and seniors cool faster, while very fit males require the highest treatment dose, due to their blunted responses to stress and extra heat generated by the muscles in the process of cooling. In addition, the perception of the same treatment differs greatly from one person to another depending on their individual tolerance limits. Consequently, these characteristics and a person's own thermal comfort level must be assessed and accounted for upon onboarding. What is barely enough cooling for a young athlete can turn out to be much too much for an overweight retiree and unimaginable for a skinny adolescent. Following the same approach across the board inevitably results in insufficient results in some cases, lack of satisfaction with the therapy in many others, and even compromised treatment safety.

The best practice is to always start with a shorter, milder session (in terms of windchill), especially if a person is new to whole body cryotherapy or has had previous experience with a different type of equipment. The first exposure can be as short as 90 seconds, and the main purpose of it is acclimatization and assessment of bodily reactions and changes in skin temperature, not a full-fledged fight-or-flight. The skin temperature drop must be sufficient yet safe. Based on the outcomes, the treatment duration, frequency, and timing can be customized, and the dose can be increased to optimize the effects of cooling. Interestingly, even the time of day of the visit to the cryotherapy center can make a difference, as body temperature and blood sugar levels fluctuate throughout the day.

Adjusting to availability and time limitations

Most of the time, the ideal cryotherapy regimen cannot be followed even if it is skillfully crafted, based on the soundest of recommendations. The limiting factors may include the travel distance to the cryotherapy location, availability only on certain days or during certain hours of the day due to work or family-related schedules, or other objective restrictions. Nevertheless, it is wise to start with the best plan and to use it as a benchmark, working around obstacles whenever possible and finding the closest alternative when not. For example, although daily treatments are likely to produce maximum gains, reducing the number to 5 or 4 days per week and, maybe, adding the second session on the most relaxed day will always be more effective than leaving the rhythm to random.

Seeking synergies with other wellness treatments

Today, most wellness centers offer more than one service and often bundle them through combination packages or "pick whatever you like" memberships. This presents a great opportunity to get more from each visit, especially because a whole body cryotherapy session is so brief. But it also increases the risks of putting the body under too much stress at once or stacking therapies that offset one another's benefits. Treatments including but not limited to whole body cryotherapy initiate a cascade of massive systemic effects, meaning that any combination must be chosen knowingly and carefully.

Whole body cryotherapy could be effectively and safely combined with, for example, light therapy, compression and lymphatic drainage, vitamin shots or intravenous infusions, and even therapies that include heat or warmth, but it is also possible to jeopardize the results or even cause health problems. Well-defined protocols and/or professional oversight are therefore required to understand implications, manage risks, and maximize the outcomes of each combination, not in general but for every individual. As already discussed, one size does not fit all.

The variables to consider include:

- The main aim of the treatment and the purpose of stacking it with other practices
- Sensibility of the combination and the potential for synergies
- Specific health considerations and individual needs

- The right dose and timing of each treatment within the combination — intensity, duration, and sequence
- Repetition requirements and a need for breaks.

If risks are understood and eliminated and synergy potential is exploited, one could use whole body cryotherapy in addition to localized and other forms of cryotherapy, all kinds of saunas including infrared, floating, hyperbaric oxygen therapy (receiving oxygen in a pressurized environment) and oxygen deprivation (altitude training), salt therapy, all kinds of massages, and much more. Some treatments, for example cryotherapy and compression, could be planned back to back, while some other combinations require more consideration — choosing an optimum sequence, spacing them out, or even doing them on alternate days. Just as it is possible to eat healthily and still overeat, it is also possible to overdose on wellness treatments.

Incorporating lifestyle adjustments

As stressed by all researchers studying the benefits of whole body cryotherapy, it can be instrumental in achieving faster progress in many situations, from inflammation and pain management to sleep and mood improvement and beyond, but it should never be seen as an isolated practice. Exposure to cold causes hormesis — the good stress that helps the body become stronger, be more resilient, and function better. So, cryotherapy will best support one's quest for improved performance, health, and longevity as a lifestyle adjustment, not as a one-time or short-term practice. Nutrition, sleep hygiene, physical activity, spending time in nature, breathwork, mindfulness exercises, and social life are among the most important aspects to mention, besides lessening the negative impacts of external factors such as air quality, noise, artificial light, and chemical and electromagnetic "pollution."

***

Chapter summary

By classification, cryotherapy falls into the category of physiotherapeutic treatments that do not cure diseases but help restore, maintain, and make the most of the person's mobility, function, and overall well-being. It is not medical and works best if incorporated into one's lifestyle as a "good stress" practice along with exercise and in addition to a nutritious diet, good-quality sleep, and mental hygiene, but the involvement of a health professional may be required to define the best treatment regimen and combination with other strategies in the case of a medical condition. While a healthy person could cryo two to three times per week on an ongoing basis, taking occasional breaks to offset habituation, tackling a health problem always requires more consideration.

Cryotherapy is well tolerated by most people regardless of age, sex, or walk of life, but the approach needs customization — there is no one universal result-producing recipe. The individual plan and the best synergistic wellness practices to supplement it should be defined based on the intended results but should also exclude risks of negative side effects and account for personal characteristics, susceptibility to cold, availability, and time limitations to maximize effectiveness without compromising safety and destroying perception. In some cases, treatment dose must be lower at first and increase gradually as the body adapts to the cold stress. In some other situations, cryotherapy may turn out not to be the right solution at all.

Researchers have come up with some general conclusions that should inform the protocol choice, for example:

The minimum number of treatments to achieve a therapeutic effect is ten sessions once daily or as often as possible, while the result will usually be better and last longer after 20 sessions in a 4-week period.

The minimum duration of a session should be 2 minutes unless its purpose is a first-time introduction to the treatment, or risks related to a medical condition have been identified. In general, exposures below 2 minutes are unlikely to produce sufficient skin temperature drop to initiate the beneficial fight-or-flight reaction on which the efficacy of whole body cryotherapy relies.

Chapter 7

What's Next? The Biohacking Road to a Better Life

The key to creating health is figuring out the cause of the problem and then providing the right conditions for the body and soul to thrive. It isn't taking another medication. The body is one integrated system, not a collection of organs divided up by medical specialties. The medicine of the future connects everything.

— Mark Hyman, MD

We live in interesting and super-dynamic times, characterized by simultaneous regress and progress, groundbreaking research findings, and major paradigm shifts.

On the one hand, we are recording the highest percentage of obese people in history and keep facing staggering statistics of diabetes, heart disease, cancer, dementia, mental illness, and suicide. The culprits of these problems are satellites of the modern lifestyle — lack of movement, poor nutrition, emotional stress overload, and the disappearance of natural physical stressors, such as having to deal with seasons-related cold versus heat, and abundance versus scarcity of food. On the other hand, we are witnessing massive developments in technology that are enabling us to learn things about the body's functioning that wouldn't be showing even in the most elaborate blood panels and, most importantly, learn how to influence them. Metabolism, insulin response, sleep quality, and the speed of biological versus chronological aging are just a few examples.

When it comes to research, age-related deterioration is increasingly classified as a disease, as it is becoming more and more evident that this process has recognizable signs and symptoms and specific causes, each of which can be reduced to a cellular and molecular level and addressed. The harmful effects of chronic low-grade inflammation have been recognized to the point where the term *inflammaging*, which was first introduced a couple of decades ago, has found a stable place in the medical professionals' vocabulary.

In the context of the above, one of the biggest paradigm shifts of the modern era is understanding that we can get actively involved in our own biology. We have a lot of control over our speed of aging and both our lifespan and our health span, collectively referred to as longevity, as the right combination of nutrition, movement, and hormesis or "good stress" can do more for the body than any drug. Consequently, we do not have to be sick and miserable in old age, falling victim to age-related diseases. We have what it takes to live to 120 or longer and remain physically capable and mentally sharp. The related practices are taught in detail by numerous scientists, doctors, and biohackers turned authors and podcasters — David Sinclair, Peter Attia, Dave Asprey, Mark Hyman, to mention just a few, are all in their fifties or even sixties and going stronger than decades earlier. Whole body cryotherapy as one of the beneficial stressors is promoted by all of them, becoming one of the treatments of the twenty-first century.

So, *what's next?*

First, thanks largely to the experiences of the recent pandemic and the "a-ha" moments related to the limitations of conventional medical care, *the new do-it-yourself biology will be adopted as a way of life by an increasing number of people.* For most "biohackers," it will not mean advanced regenerative medical practices but rather small, incremental diet or lifestyle changes. This is an easy, safe, and affordable way to wellness, as the body is built to always seek homeostasis. Using good stress, such as regular extreme cold exposure, to challenge its equilibrium results in restoring the balance at an increasingly higher level.

Then, it is finally understood that preventative wellness saves public and corporate money, and that incorporating science and technology into it can generate much better outcomes than remedies alone. *The Future of Wellness 2023 Trends* by the Global Wellness Institute clearly illustrates that wellness has become a common theme on the agendas of not only businesses serving the public but also governments, city planners, workplace wellness experts, scientists, healthcare professionals and social workers. It means that *the availability of non-medical wellness services will improve.*

Cryotherapy will keep growing in popularity in conjunction with the just-mentioned trends. The treatment has many evidence-based applications and benefits, of which reduction of systemic inflammation — the fuel of most health conditions, aging, and age-related physical and cognitive decline — is among the most researched. Studies also support balancing physical and mental state through cryotherapy. The knowledge of cryotherapy uses is spreading, and the treatment is being offered in various environments, from specialized wellness centers and exercise facilities to hotels and spas, gradually becoming an integral part of the modern lifestyle.

Understanding of the different uses of cold will deepen. Currently, the term "cryotherapy" often gets applied to all cold-based modalities without providing specifics, often leading to misunderstandings, or causing wrong expectations. As a result, it is possible that someone who expects to receive a fat-freezing treatment gets booked for whole body cryotherapy or vice versa. Hence this brief explanation:

- *Whole body cryostimulation*, which is the sole subject of this book, is only one of the current treatments involving extremely low temperatures, yet it is the most far-reaching and versatile. To some extent, especially if a cryochamber is not easily accessible, it could be replaced with an ice bath, but a plunge is a more challenging experience with less impact on the core temperature, as discussed in Chapter 1.

- When it comes to pain and swelling reduction, a store-bought or even self-made cold pack could help, but *localized cryotherapy* with a spot-cooling device powered by electricity or vapors of liquified nitrogen or carbon dioxide is more effective in less time and better controlled. All equipment in this category measures skin temperature in the application area to ensure that enough cold gets delivered without causing any tissue damage.

- Then there is the increasingly widespread body-contouring trend relying on *cryolipolysis* — targeted destruction of fat cells by lowering their temperature. These treatments, mainly of an aesthetic nature, are performed using specialized equipment to reach the subcutaneous levels of cells, which means delivering cold via contact with the skin or under significant pressure. The impact is restricted to the treatment area and cannot be achieved by whole body cryotherapy or most localized cryotherapy devices.

- Finally, we must briefly mention *cryoablation* which is a minimally invasive procedure that uses extreme cold to kill abnormal or diseased tissue, for example, tumors. Cryosurgeries are only offered in a medical setting and fall outside our conversation about non-medical wellness.

As the number of holistic wellness services that impact the body's health, performance, and appearance keeps increasing and almost every provider builds a portfolio of synergistic offerings rather than focusing on just one, we can also expect that treatment combinations will keep evolving and replacing the "pill for every ill" approach of conventional medicine. New ways of stacking services will steadily be discovered and employed on a bigger scale. One of today's "hot topics" is combining whole body cryotherapy with hyperbaric oxygen therapy (HBOT) in the context of overcoming chronic fatigue and long Covid and improving longevity, but this is just one example. There is compression and lymphatic drainage, light, oxygen, salt therapies, and many more, through which the natural pillars of health can be not only mimicked but also brought to levels inaccessible without today's modern technology.

Here are a few examples to suggest the most beneficial wellness practices that are complementary to whole body cryotherapy:

- Infrared sauna can provide the warmth of the sun that we all crave regardless of the season. It increases heart rate just like an aerobic exercise and promotes detoxification through sweating, as well as relaxing the nervous system.
- Photobiomodulation or light therapy brings the benefits of only the most powerful healing wavelengths of the sun's spectrum (depending on the device, it may be red to stimulate cell energy, infrared for pain relief and destressing, green to improve skin quality, or antibacterial blue), while excluding the harmful ultraviolet rays.
- Compression therapy and lymphatic drainage help move fluids from extremities towards the core and assist with water retention reduction, circulation, and cellular waste and toxin removal.
- Hyperbaric oxygen therapy forces cells to absorb more oxygen, which provides essential cell function support.

This effect cannot be achieved in a non-pressurized environment, only during scuba diving.

- IV drips and intramuscular vitamin shots provide nourishment and hydration and support the diet and water intake by providing micronutrients at sufficient levels, which can be difficult to supply with food alone.

None of these wellness treatments replace the need for a nutrient-rich diet and drinking enough water, exercising regularly, spending time outdoors, destressing, practicing good sleeping habits, and building healthy relationships, but they can supplement an already well-conditioned lifestyle and, in the short term, also compensate for deficiencies, keeping the doctor away. The integration of practices that support the functioning of the body as one well-oiled mechanism rather than a collection of organs is the future of health care. There is no doubt that cold therapies will be a solid part of it.

***

Chapter summary

Despite (or maybe thanks to) the highest ever numbers of people diagnosed with diabetes, obesity, heart disease, cancer, and dementia, we are witnessing major breakthroughs and paradigm shifts in what it takes to live not only a longer but also a healthier life. It has become clear that we have much more control over our own biology and aging than we ever thought possible. A combination of nutrition, movement, and hormesis can do more for the body than any drug, and cryotherapy falls into the "good stress" category.

In the years to come, biohacking will keep becoming a way of life for increasing numbers of people. The availability of non-medical wellness services will also improve through hotels, workplaces, and governments. Whole body cryotherapy will keep growing in popularity and be integrated into the modern lifestyle, in line with a deepening understanding of other applications of cold. And synergistic treatment combinations will keep evolving to provide truly functional health care to replace today's conventional "sick care." A new era of wellness is upon us, and the future looks brighter than ever for those seeking longevity.

Epilogue

As practitioners and ambassadors of holistic drug-free wellness, we see the future in bright colors.

We consider ourselves blessed to have access to the new knowledge and technologies capable of delivering inflammation and pain reduction, energy boost, sleep improvement, and much slower biological aging to support living better for longer and, most importantly, to be able to see the fruit of it all through improving the lives of thousands of people whom we have helped embrace whole body cryotherapy.

We participate in reinventing cool and changing mindsets. But this book is not the end of our journey. It's not even the beginning of the end. It's just the end of the beginning. There is much more to do to spread the word, open eyes, and build a community of people who share our belief that, in the words of the Iceman Wim Hof, "Cold is a doorway to the soul." Regardless of where you stand in your wellness journey and whether you make cryotherapy accessible to others or only use it for your own benefit, we hope that this book, the additional resources that it leads to, and other work that we have done so far gives you the impetus to keep going and to reach new heights.

We truly believe in having a handle on our physical abilities and mental acumen for as many years as we have left to live, so that even the ripest old age is free of frailty and suffering. In our fifties, we both practice what we preach. The optimization of physical and mental wellness through cutting-edge technologies and treatment protocols and feeling, looking, performing at one's best at any age is what we stand for. It is the future of wellness to which we are committed in our personal and professional lives. Thank you for joining us on this rewarding path!

Additional Resources

We intended this book to be a quick and easy read that highlights only the most important aspects of understanding whole body cryotherapy, from the physiological reactions induced by exposing the body to extreme cold, to their benefits, possible risks, and the factors to consider in the process of building a safe and effective treatment regimen, customized to the individual's needs and goals. We hope it will help you better navigate the maze of options. At the same time, we had to limit the depth of explanation in many cases and leave some topics completely uncovered, especially when it comes to wellness as a business. For more information, use the additional resources provided on **reinventing.cool**, follow us on social media, and benefit from joining our communities.

As the preferred wellness and recovery destination for many Londoners, LondonCryo keeps accumulating case studies and success stories, many of which get shared through articles on **londoncryo.com/blog** and **linkedin.com/company/londoncryo**, as well as on a podcast hosted by Maria: Reinventing Cool at **londoncryo.com/podcasts** and LondonCryo YouTube channel. These resources will provide valuable insights if you use cryotherapy solely for your own health and wellness.

If you are a cryotherapy provider, you may look into taking the training course "The Fundamentals of Whole Body Cryotherapy" and using other wellness business oriented resources available through **getresultsco.com**. We also invite you to join the Cryotherapy and Wellness Professionals Group on Facebook for continuous education and in-depth sharing of knowledge and experiences with fellow business owners.

What Makes a Perfect Whole Body Cryotherapy Session

When it comes to arranging the initial cryotherapy appointment, many first-timers tend to get unnecessarily anxious. As a rule of thumb, cold environments are not perceived as comfortable, and standing half-naked in a cabin in which the temperature is around –100°C, even if only for a few minutes, sounds scary. If a cold shower feels bad, how can anyone survive such extremely cold air?

For most people, to their great surprise, the actual experience does not feel bad at all, largely because cold air withdraws heat from the body much more slowly than water, but proper preparation is the make-or-break factor for both sides — the treatment provider and the user. Let us outline the elements of it.

The first step must always be filling out the intake questionnaire and looking into any responses that stand out. This should not be seen as an unnecessary formality or nosiness on the center's part because, as discussed, whole body cryotherapy may present certain risks to some people. The contraindications, if any, must be excluded. In some cases, a physician may have to be consulted to establish whether trying cryotherapy is a good idea. It is also highly recommended to avoid whole body cryotherapy if you notice any signs of a cold, weakness, or dizziness, as the cold shock may amplify the discomfort.

If no obstacles have been identified, once the intake documentation is complete and before the first treatment can take place, elucidation of what happens during the cryotherapy session and setting accurate expectations is extremely important.

In addition to the specifics of the site, equipment, and intended application, this includes the following:

- A general description of the treatment process, including the expected physiological reactions and sensations.
- Instruction to keep breathing relaxed, flat, and slow. Feeling a little pressure in the chest is normal, as air is denser in the cold environment and expands once inhaled.
- Instruction to stand still or move fluidly. Rapid movements should be avoided, as they increase air flow and speed up cooling in the affected areas, which may lead to overcooling. Leaning against or touching the chamber walls, on the other hand, may lead to an immediate case of frostbite.
- Instruction to cover the area of the body that feels too cold with a gloved hand. This usually applies to the thinner skin around the elbows.
- Instruction to step out of the cryochamber at any time if feeling uncomfortable or noticing any unusual sensation besides tingling.
- Warning to watch the step when coming out of the cryochamber to avoid tripping or slipping, as the floor may be uneven, the soles of your shoes may have hardened in the cold environment, and there may be some frost on the floor.

If some nervousness remains, a few slow breaths before proceeding, or seeing someone else do the treatment first, may help relieve the stress.

Preparation for the session includes a few routine steps, including:

- Making sure that all clothes that will be worn while inside the chamber (underwear, shorts, bra) are sufficiently warm, completely dry, and without any metal parts touching the skin.

- Putting on the mandatory protective gear of the acral areas in which concentration of nerve endings and therefore sensitivity is very high. This includes cotton or wool socks, shoes with thick soles, gloves, a headband or a cap to cover ears and parts of the head without hair, and a face mask.
- Making sure that the skin is dry and free of lotions, creams, or oils. Any excess liquid may freeze in the sub-zero temperatures and cause irritation or frostbite.
- Making sure that all large accessories that may get too cold during the session are taken off and left in the changing room.

Having eaten prior to WBC or coming from a workout does not present a problem, but showering right before or after is neither recommended nor necessary.

Since the comfort level of the cold exposure depends on many individual characteristics, including but not limited to susceptibility to cold, and even previous experiences, it is better to start with a shorter or milder trial session and test the body's reactions during the treatment and in the few hours that follow. Based on the findings, next time the dose of cold can be increased slowly and gradually or all at once.

***

A sample treatment process

At LondonCryo, each visit begins at the reception desk by checking in with a wellness coordinator and being escorted to a changing room. The protective clothing readily available in the changing room includes long socks, boots, and gloves. A bath robe is also provided, for privacy.

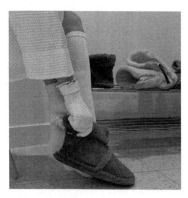

Preparing for the Session

Once ready, it is time to proceed to the treatment room.

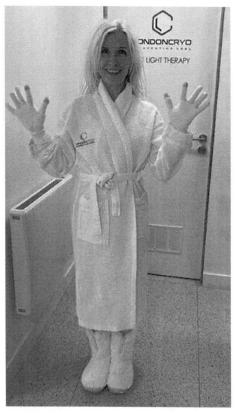

Ready for Treatment

The cryocabin at LondonCryo is cooled by injecting liquid nitrogen vapors into its cylindrical open-top treatment space. To avoid wasting any time, it is first pre-cooled to –110°C. Once the target temperature has been reached, the wellness coordinator opens the door and the client enters the cabin, then removes the robe and passes it to the operator. The session begins and is supervised till the end.

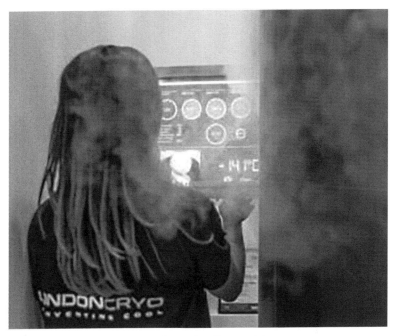

Precooling the Cryocabin

During the 3-minute session, the temperature of the cold, dry vapor encircling the client continues to go down until it reaches approximately –130°C to –140°C. Nitrogen gas is heavier than air and stays below the chin level. The person inside breathes regular room-temperature air and can communicate with the operator throughout the session. The staff member in charge makes sure that the client feels comfortable and needs no assistance.

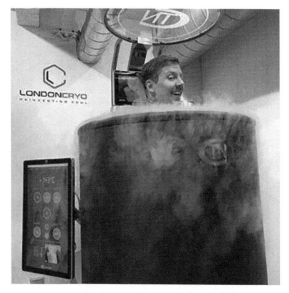

Treatment in Progress

Once the countdown timer signals that the session is over, the client is handed back their robe, exits the cabin, and returns to the changing room unless scheduled for another service. The post-session endorphin rush and blood circulation boost leaves people energized and in a good mood.

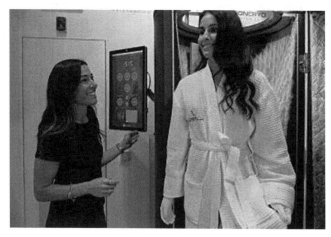

End of the Treatment

Appendix 2

Most Frequently Asked Questions

- *What is whole body cryotherapy (WBC) in a nutshell?*
  Whole body cryotherapy is the brief and safe exposure of the entire body to extremely low temperatures, usually around –100°C, that the body perceives as dangerous; in response, it engages the most potent mechanisms to keep the core temperature from dropping. This so-called fight-or-flight reaction involves beneficial responses including but not limited to blood circulation boost, release of natural painkillers and mood lifters (endorphins), and activation of the parasympathetic nervous system.

- *Is cryotherapy just a technologically more advanced ice bath?*
  There are similarities but also a few major differences that make WBC and ice baths complementary rather than substitutive for one another. WBC triggers the protective fight-or-flight reaction within seconds and draws blood to the core, supplying oxygen and nutrients to all essential organs and keeping the core warm. Only the skin temperature is affected, and reaping the benefits takes just a few minutes of exposure. Physical activity can be planned immediately after the WBC session, since the influx of energy and muscle oxygenation provides extra power to move. Cold water immersion requires between 10 and 20 minutes to be therapeutic. In such a long time, cold begins to penetrate the subcutaneous tissue and reaches the muscles, stiffening them and temporarily reducing mobility. The modality is great

for pain management and muscle recovery, but not for performance enhancement, and its impact on the organs surrounding the core is less pronounced.

- *Isn't cryotherapy only for professional athletes?*
  While many professional athletes do take advantage of whole body cryotherapy benefits that include performance boost, injury prevention, and faster recovery post-exertion, there are many more applications. Initially, the modality was developed for the purposes of arthritis pain management. Since the late 1970s when it was born, many more indications have been added, including but not limited to back and neck pains of various kinds, ankylosing spondylitis, fibromyalgia, multiple sclerosis, tendinopathies, skin conditions, and mood and sleep disorders.

- *How can a human being withstand temperatures below −100°C?*
  It is possible thanks to the super-effective thermoregulatory system of the human body. There is an ongoing communication between the thermoreceptors in the skin and the temperature control center in the brain. As soon as a discrepancy is detected, heat production is either down-regulated to cool or up-regulated to support the optimal functioning of all organs and systems. The extreme temperatures inside the cryochamber would lead to hypothermia in the long run, but the session is timed so that the skin temperature over the cold exposure does not fall below 4°C. The drop is sufficient to initiate the beneficial fight-or-flight reaction yet remains within safe limits. If all treatment-related instructions are properly followed, no damage occurs.

• *Does a cryotherapy session hurt?*

Depending on the person's cold sensitivity, the cold may feel uncomfortable to some extent, but it does not hurt and feels much better than most first-timers expect. Although the temperatures inside a cryochamber are much lower than even the coldest water, the sensation is less extreme because the air is dry and withdraws heat more than 20 times more slowly than water. For this same reason, +20°C air feels like summer while +20°C lake water would be considered too cold to swim by many. Closer to the end of the 3-minute exposure, the skin may start tingling, but there is no actual freezing involved and no tissue gets damaged, and most people don't even shiver. Those who do are advised to begin with shorter treatments and acclimatize gradually. If the cold feels too much, the session can be stopped at any time.

• *Why is it necessary to take cryotherapy treatment with minimal clothing?*

Since cryotherapy relies on the body's reaction to the extremely low temperatures it uses, it is essential that the skin surface with its cold sensors is maximally exposed. Every piece of clothing that is left on blunts the responses and reduces the efficacy of the treatment. There are just a few exceptions: the feet and, particularly, the toes, fingertips, and genitalia in men. The concentration of nerve endings in these areas is simply too high to bear the cold for the required 3 minutes. In addition, while undergoing cryotherapy, the body pulls blood away from the extremities and into the core, so the acral areas must have extra protection. Socks, gloves, and underwear are therefore required and should be completely dry, sufficiently thick, and, preferably, contain cotton or wool.

- *Could I catch a cold from using cryotherapy?*
  This should not happen due to the protective reactions that the body engages in response to whole body cryotherapy. Cryotherapy enhances blood flow and is proven to cause anti-inflammatory and antioxidant chemical reactions. The "good stress," or hormesis, unless overdosed, improves the body's resilience and strengthens the immune system, so it may even decrease the severity and frequency of future colds and susceptibility to viruses. At the same time, undergoing cryotherapy when already feeling sick would be counterproductive. Cough, congestion, or fever should be taken as signs to let the body rest. It is already experiencing stress, and increasing the load may worsen the symptoms rather than relieve them.

- *How should I prepare for my whole body cryotherapy treatment? Should I shower before or after?*
  No special preparation is required. Cryotherapy is easy to squeeze into the daily schedule; it takes very little time and can be done even during the lunch break. Eating or exercising right before or after the session is not a problem. Most centers provide all necessary gear. It just needs to be remembered that the procedure requires the skin and everything on it to be completely dry. All water, sweat, and body lotions, creams, or oils, if used, should be wiped off with a dry towel before entering the cryochamber. Showering is neither required nor recommended, as any residual moisture that's left on the body could lead to frostbite. Extreme caution should be exercised if cryotherapy is combined with any treatment that involves heat and causes perspiration.

- *What should I expect from cryotherapy treatment?*
  To answer this question, we should distinguish between the exposure itself and the hours following it.

  During the session, depending on the technology in use, the body is surrounded by either very cold air or vapors of liquid nitrogen. The nitrogen-powered devices leave the head outside, while the electric chambers look and feel like walk-in freezers. While inside, the cold makes the skin temperature drop. It feels chilly but bearable. The treatment is short, and the best approach is to breathe slowly and evenly and to relax as much as possible, thinking of the benefits that the body is reaping. The skin may tingle a bit. Slight shivering closer to the end of the session is also possible yet not very common.

  Upon exiting, if there was any pain, it may have disappeared. This happens thanks to the analgesic powers of cold — it slows pain signal transmission and reduces pain sensitivity. A feeling of happiness that many characterize as a "natural high" sets in as the body celebrates its escape from the extreme environment. This feeling is caused by the release of endorphins. As the blood starts returning to the peripherals, the body feels an influx of energy. These effects can last for several hours post-session, while the intangible improvements accumulate gradually, just as they do from regular exercise or positive diet changes. To achieve sustainable results, just one cryotherapy session is never enough.

- *Can I derive benefits from just one session?*
  The immediate benefits include pain relief and a boost in mood and energy. Many people report sleeping better the following night. Blood tests show antioxidant and

anti-inflammatory chemical reactions. But, without committing to a series of sessions that science proves to be at least ten, these improvements will be short-lived.

- *If I exercise, should I do cryotherapy before or after?*
  Either or even both! The best timing depends on the intended outcome. Cryotherapy before exercise or a sporting event may heighten both physical and mental performance by improving blood flow throughout the body, including the brain, oxygenation of the muscles, optimizing the energy budget, and reducing pain sensitivity. The expected outcomes are more energy and stamina, less pain, and less sweating. Cryotherapy after athletic exertion may help with inflammation and soreness reduction and restoration of the depleted energy reserve. Studies show significantly faster recovery if whole body cryotherapy is involved.

- *Has whole body cryotherapy been proven as a recovery modality?*
  The use of cryotherapy for athletic performance and recovery has been studied much more than for any other application, resulting in many publications and recommendations for use. Refer to **reinventing.cool/proof** for the findings.

- *How often should I do cryotherapy?*
  It is recommended to commit to at least ten cryotherapy sessions in the first 30 days for optimal results, while in a post-surgery or post-injury phase even a few consecutive treatments could substantially reduce the inflammation and swelling. Depending on the condition, especially if lessening of the symptoms of a medical condition is

desired, it may be beneficial to maximize the frequency to five to seven treatments per week until noticeable improvement is achieved. For maintenance, two to three exposures per week have proven to be sufficient.

- *Should I see a doctor before the first treatment?*
Cryotherapy is a non-medical "wellness for all" type of therapy that has been proven to deliver many benefits, including but not limited to enhanced recovery, reduced inflammation and pain, more energy, and better sleep. Seeing a doctor would only be recommended, or sometimes even required, in the case of a medical condition that is considered a contraindication, especially those that impair the cardiovascular system. Cryotherapy temporarily increases the heart rate and systolic blood pressure and boosts circulation, which benefits healthy individuals but could cause too much stress for people with heart disease, hypertension, blood clots, or damaged blood vessels. You will find a full list of conditions that are considered somewhat risky in our resource portal. To review, visit **reinventing.cool/contraindications**. Before the first treatment, every user is required to disclose their health concerns and sign a liability waiver, taking responsibility for the consequences. In case of any doubts, consulting a medical professional is strongly encouraged.

- *Can whole body cryotherapy be used by claustrophobic people?*
Claustrophobia is seen as a relative contraindication. The answer depends on the severity of the condition and the equipment in use. People who are afraid of closed spaces may want to choose a head-outside cryosauna rather than a walk-in cryochamber. In cryosaunas, the head remains above the upper edge of the cabin, and the operator is

always there, observing, communicating, and ready to help, if necessary. Also, the door is never locked, and the treatment can be stopped at any moment.

- *I am pregnant; can I do whole body cryotherapy?*
  Whole body cryotherapy is a thermal shock treatment and, for obvious reasons, its effects on the fetus have not been studied. During pregnancy, it is best to exclude all possible risks and to avoid experiments with the unknown. Cryotherapy should therefore be avoided.

- *Why should I spend money on something like this?*
  People rarely realize how much living in pain costs them, not to mention debilitating health conditions that come with other symptoms such as chronic fatigue, brain fog, or insomnia, and the toll that they take not only physically but also emotionally. Let's look at the statistics. "Sick care" is expensive. On average, one American who suffers from chronic pain spends about $6000 per year on pain-related medications and manipulations alone. Another $6000, or more, is lost because of lower productivity. Besides, most pain medications are designed to mask symptoms, not to eliminate the cause, and have side effects, especially if taken regularly. One pill per day today leads to three in the foreseeable future and dependence on prescription drugs for life. If the cause is inflammation of any kind, cryotherapy (and some other nature-based holistic practices) may be the best and one of the least costly investments in living a pain-free life again and enjoying all it brings. And pain relief is just one of the many outcomes that could be achieved.

Appendix 3

The Results Speak for Themselves

To give a few examples of what can be expected, below are some quotes from people who have turned to cryotherapy for various reasons.

A woman with arthritis:

> I came a month ago with extreme pain and now, after a month of whole body cryotherapy, I feel much better than before. I would highly recommend WBC if you have suffered from arthritis and problems with joints, and it is a great stress reliever.

A man who could not walk after a fall:

> After falling from the top of my stairs, I thought I was never going to walk normally again. I tripped at the beginning of the stairs one morning after rushing out of my bedroom because I heard the fire alarm. In stress, I ended up breaking my hip bone, went through a surgery, and started physiotherapy after, but my recovery process was extremely slow, and walking was excruciatingly painful. Little by little, I was able to walk again, but it was never the same as before. A friend of mine told me about cryotherapy, and, out of desperation, I decided to go for a session. To be honest, all I felt at first was cold; I didn't think there was anything happening. But I was encouraged to go for more sessions while still undergoing physiotherapy, and I noticed that walking was becoming easier. It has been 3 years now, and I walk as I used to

before the fall. I'm grateful I tried it out. It was the best decision I have ever made in my life. I will forever be grateful to the inventors of cryotherapy.

A man with a chronic skin lesion:

I started noticing some strange papules on my skin, and I felt maybe it was just an allergic reaction. But the next day I was shocked to see that what I observed the previous day had doubled in size, and there were new papules on other parts of my body. They kept on increasing, and about 3 days later I decided to go to the hospital. I was told I had an autoimmune disease, then some other symptoms followed. My issue wasn't with the other symptoms because they were managed, but the skin lesion reduction was extremely slow. It covered my whole arm and neck, and I felt embarrassed to leave the house. One day I was in the hospital for my checkup and complained to my doctor about the lesion. He prescribed some medications, but also suggested I try out cryotherapy. Following my doctor's advice, I went ahead and booked a session. After several treatments, the lesion started reducing. I still have a bit of it left, but after about 2 months of consistent cryotherapy I can see a significant change.

A medical doctor with a history of various sports injuries:

As a medical doctor I wanted to try this cutting-edge technology firsthand. I had been focusing on my sports recovery since I suffered from various injuries, but I can honestly say that this addition to my recovery has helped in many ways. I now come on average three to four times per week and combine whole body cryo with compression therapy and localized cryotherapy. I also do infrared sauna and photobiomodulation. Since incorporating it all into my physical and mental wellness journey, I am the fittest I've ever been. After all, the best investment you can make is in yourself.

A man with a severe knee inflammation:

I have had three knee operations and have severe damage to my meniscus on my left knee. It has been inflamed for several years and I've tried everything to fix it, from stem cell surgery to numerous physio programs. After just 3 weeks of cryotherapy, my knee has completely recovered, and the inflammation has disappeared. Incredible results from three sessions a week! I am over the moon I discovered this practice and recommend this for anyone with damaged knee cartilage or meniscus tears.

A man with a long history of back pain:

I have been dealing with low back pain for years. Almost every morning I would have to take a pain medication just to ease the pain and to perform normally both at my job and weight training. And then cryotherapy changed it all. I have had a total of five sessions so far, and my lower back has never felt this great! I not only feel extremely energized after every session, but I'm also gaining my low-back strength back. Oh, and did I mention that I have completely discontinued taking pain meds?

A woman with pins and needles in her arms from a pinched nerve:

I have had a trapped nerve in my neck for several months, which was causing pins and needles and loss of strength in my arms. The doctor referred me to a physio, but results were very slow. I was aware of cryotherapy and asked to try one session. It was amazingly effective, and I was pain-free for over a week. My physio who saw me shortly after that was amazed that the vertebrae in my neck appeared to be working perfectly. After the second session it improved again and, having had the third session to alleviate tension across my shoulders, the neck is pain-free, the pins and needles have stopped, and the strength is returning to my hands. Brilliant treatment and fabulous results!

A woman suffering from lasting nerve damage and having trouble sleeping:

I have been using cryotherapy for 9 months and it has changed my life. I have been in pain management for 18 years for nerve damage. My pain was getting worse, and the doctor wanted to increase my pain medication once again, but I didn't want to be on anything stronger. I started cryotherapy, have not had to change my medication, and have not had any more pain. I also had to take an over-the-counter antihistamine tablet to help me sleep at least four times a week. I have not taken any since starting treatment. I sleep so well every night. I would recommend it to anyone with any type of pain.

Perri Shakes-Drayton, Team GB Olympian:

My experience of using cryotherapy is very positive. Unlike after an ice bath, I can train following the 3-minute session. I've benefited from cryotherapy from a recovery aspect after a long week of training, and I've also used it before, both of which have helped bring the best out in me. Once the session is complete, it gives me a feel-good factor and leaves my skin silky smooth.

@faisalPmAfitness, one of the UK's biggest fitness influencers:

I've been doing a weekly session for the past 5 weeks, as I've upped my training ahead of a triathlon. Putting my body into flight-or-fight mode at a temperature of –130°C every week has allowed me to train harder with more intensity and volume. I'll definitely be carrying on with my sessions post-triathlon. I'm hooked!

To conclude, we will quote a woman who has been struggling with shoulder pain for years. After several sessions of cryotherapy at LondonCryo, she was asked to write down ten things to summarize her experience. Here is what she wrote:

1. I feel more energized.
2. The pain I used to have is no more.
3. I feel better and more at peace with myself.
4. My relationships are better. The shoulder pain affected my ability to function effectively as a wife to my husband and as a mother to my children.
5. I have improved greatly at work. My boss even gave me a promotion.
6. I feel a general state of improved well-being.
7. I think cryotherapy is not spoken about enough; the world needs to know this miracle.
8. I've recommended cryotherapy to my extended family members and friends, and those who tried it have noticed great improvements.
9. Cryotherapy is the best.
10. If I had enough resources, I would have started my own cryotherapy center.

Acknowledgments

No one achieves their dream alone.

This book would not be possible without the people in our lives: our families, co-workers, clients, and the diverse and purpose-driven community of wellness center owners and equipment providers with whom we get to exchange resources and experiences daily.

Our most sincere thanks go to our partners Antonie Iannello and Hilko De Brouwer for believing in us and supporting our endeavors and to the team at LondonCryo for being part of the process from day one.

We must also acknowledge the long list of people who have contributed to raising awareness of the benefits of cold and promoting whole body cryotherapy as a wellness and recovery tool. Scientists and educators like David Sinclair and Andrew Huberman. Medical doctors and authors like Peter Attia and Mark Hyman. Biohacking entrepreneurs and public figures like Tony Robbins, Dave Asprey, and Ben Greenfield. Trailblazers and challengers of what's possible like Wim Hof. Hard-working superstar athletes like LeBron James. And the list goes on. Thanks to them, people have started taking responsibility for their health and well-being in an all-new way, and we could not be prouder to put in our two cents.

Disclaimer

This book and the additional materials referenced in it, as well as the websites and any appearances of the authors on social or other media, are for general information purposes only.

While hundreds of studies on the effects of whole body cryotherapy have already been conducted, the extreme cold exposures remain a beneficial non-medical adjunct approach to a stronger, better-functioning body rather than a stand-alone solution to any health, performance, or recovery-related problem. The United States Food and Drug Administration (FDA) or its counterparts in other countries have not evaluated the statements made throughout this book and the supporting resources. The materials that we have brought to you are based solely on our own research, experiences, and opinions. No statement is intended to diagnose, treat, cure, or prevent any disease. No recommendation can replace professional advice or should be seen as a discouragement to seek such advice.

In the case of any preexisting condition, we strongly recommend consulting the doctor in charge and getting their explicit consent and protocol suggestion for incorporating cryotherapy into the treatment regimen. Any decision based on this input is made at the user's own risk and is their own responsibility.

O-BOOKS

SPIRITUALITY

O is a symbol of the world, of oneness and unity; this eye represents knowledge and insight. We publish titles on general spirituality and living a spiritual life. We aim to inform and help you on your own journey in this life.
If you have enjoyed this book, why not tell other readers by posting a review on your preferred book site?

Recent bestsellers from O-Books are:

Heart of Tantric Sex
Diana Richardson
Revealing Eastern secrets of deep love and intimacy to Western couples.
Paperback: 978-1-90381-637-0 ebook: 978-1-84694-637-0

Crystal Prescriptions
The A–Z guide to over 1,200 symptoms and their healing crystals
Judy Hall
The first in the popular series of eight books, this handy little guide is packed as tight as a pill bottle with crystal remedies for ailments.
Paperback: 978-1-90504-740-6 ebook: 978-1-84694-629-5

Shine On
David Ditchfield and J S Jones
What if the after effects of a near-death experience were
undeniable? What if a person could suddenly produce
high-quality paintings of the afterlife, or if they
acquired the ability to compose classical symphonies?
Meet: David Ditchfield.
Paperback: 978-1-78904-365-5 ebook: 978-1-78904-366-2

The Way of Reiki
The Inner Teachings of Mikao Usui
Frans Stiene
The roadmap for deepening your understanding
of the system of Reiki and rediscovering
your True Self.
Paperback: 978-1-78535-665-0 ebook: 978-1-78535-744-2

You Are Not Your Thoughts
Frances Trussell
The journey to a mindful way of being, for those who want
to truly know the power of mindfulness.
Paperback: 978-1-78535-816-6 ebook: 978-1-78535-817-3

The Mysteries of the Twelfth Astrological House
Fallen Angels
Carmen Turner-Schott, MSW, LISW
Everyone wants to know more about the most misunderstood
house in astrology — the twelfth astrological house.
Paperback: 978-1-78099-343-0 ebook: 978-1-78099-344-7

WhatsApps from Heaven
Louise Hamlin

An account of a bereavement and the extraordinary
signs — including WhatsApps — that a retired
law lecturer received from her deceased husband.

Paperback: 978-1-78904-947-3 ebook: 978-1-78904-948-0

The Holistic Guide to Your Health
& Wellbeing Today
Oliver Rolfe

A holistic guide to improving your complete health,
both inside and out.

Paperback: 978-1-78535-392-5 ebook: 978-1-78535-393-2

Cool Sex
Diana Richardson and Wendy Doeleman

For deeply satisfying sex, the real secret is to reduce the heat,
to cool down. Discover the empowerment and fulfilment
of sex with loving mindfulness.

Paperback: 978-1-78904-351-8 ebook: 978-1-78904-352-5

Creating Real Happiness A to Z
Stephani Grace

Creating Real Happiness A to Z will help you understand
the truth that you are not your ego
(conditioned self).

Paperback: 978-1-78904-951-0 ebook: 978-1-78904-952-7

A Colourful Dose of Optimism

Jules Standish

It's time for us to look on the bright side, by boosting
our mood and lifting our spirit, both in
our interiors, as well as in our closet.
Paperback: 978-1-78904-927-5 ebook: 978-1-78904-928-2

Readers of ebooks can buy or view any of these bestsellers by
clicking on the live link in the title. Most titles are published
in paperback and as an ebook. Paperbacks are available in
traditional bookshops. Both print and ebook formats are
available online.

Find more titles and sign up to our readers' newsletter at
www.o-books.com

Follow O-Books on Facebook at **O-Books**

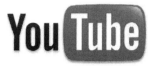

For video content, author interviews and more, please subscribe to our YouTube channel:

O-BOOKS Presents

Follow us on social media for book news, promotions and more:

Facebook: O-Books

Instagram: @o_books_mbs

X: @obooks

Tik Tok: @ObooksMBS

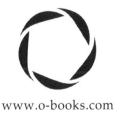

www.o-books.com